EMOTIONAL EATING

How to Stop Overeating and Binge Eating. Feed Your Feelings and Improve Relationship with Food

JESSICA LANE

Table of Contents

Introduction

What is emotional eating?

When emotional eating is discussed in medical contexts, it refers to situations in which an individual consumes unusually large amounts of food. It isn't simply the amount of food that defines these events as emotional eating, however. It's the drive behind the event—these individuals aren't motivated by extreme hunger, authentic or otherwise.

They're motivated by their emotional state. They also tend to gravitate towards foods that aren't healthy in large amounts, i.e. junk food or comfort food. Some experts believe as much as 75% of overeating events are caused by the emotional state of the individual involved.

Emotional Eating: Quick Facts

•   Eating in response to your emotions, especially but not limited to negative emotional states such as stress, sadness, and anger, rather than because you are hungry is emotional eating. Think about the movie trope regarding women eating cheesecake or ice cream when a distressing event happens in their lives. While having a treat to "cheer up" isn't necessarily a bad thing, eating excessively due to your emotional state can quickly become a pattern hard to break.

•	Most people gravitate toward foods high in carbohydrates (glucose, starches, etc.), high in calories, and low in overall nutritional value when they emotionally eat.

•	Binge eating and emotional eating can be related, and may even overlap, but there are distinctions between the two. Binge eating is defined almost entirely by the quantity of food the person is eating. Emotional eating is defined by the reason behind eating the food. You may binge when you emotionally eat; you may not. Emotions may be a primary factor in binge eating, but then again, they might not be.

•	Emotional eating isn't always (and in fact, usually is not) a single-factor issue. There are usually many contributing factors in a severe emotional eating habit.

•	Emotional eating can be identified by a number of warning signs, which we will discuss further on in this book.

- If you work with your doctor, nutritionist, or other health professional with regards to your emotional eating habits, they will take into account both physical and psychological issues when forming a treatment plan. This can help you overcome the habit of emotional eating sooner.

- In order to overcome emotional eating, you will have to reassess the way you view food. You'll have to actively develop more mindful eating habits. You'll also work to identify situational triggers that result in your emotional eating. Finally, you'll develop coping mechanisms that help you respond to these triggers in healthier ways that don't involve emotional eating. You will also learn preventative measures to help you avoid and mitigate the emotional stressors that lead to emotional eating.

- Emotional eating is a serious problem. While it is often treated lightly in media and society as a whole, it is a serious contributor to obesity, weight loss issues, eating disorders, and food addiction. By combating emotional eating, you are doing one of the best possible things you can do for yourself. Don't trivialize your journey!

- During your journey to gain autonomy over your eating habits, you'll work to reduce stress in your life in a holistic way, which has numerous benefits beyond helping you eat in a healthier manner. You'll also learn more constructive ways to address intense emotions, which can also be a fantastic way to improve your quality of life.

The issues with emotional eating go far, far beyond what you order in a restaurant or which drive-thru you choose on your way home from work. A holistic approach to emotional eating has the potential to improve your life in ways you never thought possible.

Chapter 1: Mindless Eating and Why We Do It

Eating mindlessly can cause anyone to eat way too much and this is what happens to most of us. The problem is that when people are eating, they are hardly thinking about what they are doing. Instead, their minds are on other things and this leads them to not be aware of how much they are eating. Connected to this is the fact that most people also eat while doing other things. Eating becomes a mindless act that is often done alongside watching TV or while talking with friends and in the end, much more is consumed than if the person is fully aware of what and how much he is eating.

There are many reasons why we eat mindlessly, so let's take a look at a few of these reasons below:

Availability

One of the biggest reasons we eat without thinking about how much we are eating is because the food is available. When you are sitting on the couch, you're not paying attention to what you're eating; you are paying attention to the movie, the chips are right in front of you, so you keep eating them simply because they are there.

Feelings

We often eat in order to numb any negative feelings we have, such as anger, sadness, and frustration. This is a popular coping mechanism which helps people believe they feel better about whatever negativity has affected them. We also eat because of many other feelings we have, such as feeling bored, lonely, or we are trying to avoid something.

If we suffer from anxiety, we are more likely to eat because anxiety can often make us feel that we are hungry. Some people feel that eating helps them cope with anxiety, so whenever they feel anxious, they are going to turn to food.

Boredom

People eat when they are bored, and this happens a lot. One of the main reasons why people overeat is because they have nothing to do, leading them to eating which is the most convenient and easy act. When people are at home and have nothing to do, it is easy for them to open the fridge or grab a snack from the pantry. Even when going outside, eating is one of the most popular activities that people find themselves doing when they want something to do. Eating can be done almost anywhere and at any time of the day, and many people will find that a lot of their time is spent doing so.

Stress and Anxiety

Stress and anxiety are among the top reasons why people overeat. When a person is frustrated or is faced with problems and anxieties, food becomes a default solution. Not that it solves the problem, but eating does give a sense of relief and security.

Coping with Emotions

In relation to coping with stress and anxiety, overeating is also often caused by other strong feelings or emotion. Those who are depressed, for example, find themselves drowning their sorrows in dishes of food. On the other hand, even those who are elated find themselves celebrating over huge servings of food.

For Comfort

The term 'comfort food' is not just something to persuade people to eat. For most people, there is nothing more comforting than a serving or two of their favorite dishes. Eating for comfort is very common as food gives feelings of satiation, well-being, and of course happiness.

Out of Habit

Eating is a part of life and is needed for survival; but most of the time, people eat simply out of habit. While it is just right that we eat on a regular basis, there are times when people eat just because they are used to doing so. People eat after waking up, during all their breaks at school or at work or simply when they find food or when they have nothing else to do. Like the other reasons why people overeat, eating, because of habit, is mindless and not a necessity.

Socialization

Food is almost always at the center of social situations and for this reason, many people find themselves eating more than they should. When out with friends or when celebrating special occasions, food is always sure to be involved. There are also many events where food is part of the equation. Parties always present tables filled with foods, the movies always bring popcorn and snacks, and even the workplace is filled with finger foods, coffee and drinks, or that nearby food chain where employees are sure to spend a lot of their time.

Childhood Conditioning

One further point I would like to talk about is how your childhood eating habits affect your current overeating problem.

Children are taught, are you most likely were too, that food is a reward. It is no wonder they think this as unhealthy food is given to children as a reward for good behavior, an accomplishment, a birthday, a vacation etc. This is called conditioning and conditioning is extremely hard to break especially when it begins as early as infancy. It goes even further than that though. For example, if a newborn baby cries one of the first reactions is to feed the baby; it must be hungry. Then when the baby gets older the parents take him/her to get ice cream after doing well in the school play. The child's birthday parties, and their friend's parties are another excuse to eat cake and ice cream. Weddings and even funerals are used as an excuse to overeat or to eat unhealthy foods.

Tired and Deprived

People eat because they are tired and while this only sounds logical, there are times when tiredness leads them to eat even when they are not hungry. Food becomes a pick-me-up tool that helps people get over their tiredness. However, tiredness is not the same as hunger and while food may provide a temporary solution, it can also lead to weight gain and other health problems related to overeating.

Food Everywhere

Overeating is simple to do simply because there is food everywhere. There is food inside the house, food stalls in almost every street and food chains in almost every corner. There are even food vendors who come to you so that you do not even have to look for food yourself. The result is people eat even when they do not need to simply because food is there.

Cravings

Cravings are among the top reasons why people overeat. There are times when people simply feel the need to consume certain types of food. In most cases, we cannot even explain these urges, but they are there. You may crave for a burger or a hot fudge sundae, or a nice big juicy steak. Whatever your craving is, the effect is for you to eat more than you need to and oftentimes, you will eat even more just because you are unable to get what it is you are craving for.

Chapter 2: The Psychology of Emotional Eating

When we improve on the types of foods we consume, we will most likely be able to control certain involuntary impulses and cravings, and manage our weight better. Did you know the way your day plays out is determined by what you eat? *You really are what you eat.* That's not just a cliché. It's true.

When you do not eat enough or you consume too much food, it can seriously affect your health and your way of life. This might paint a morbid image of food in your mind, but don't let it. Remember, balance is key. That's why people are less likely to eat foods which have caused them to vomit. A person is less likely to retry the food for fear of repeating the experience.

Who's the Boss? Your Head, or Your Stomach?

You have to be in control of your body and your mind. You have to be the dominant character when making food choices and not your feelings. When you are in control, you are more likely to make an effort to cut back on foods you know present a serious risk to your health.

If you leave your feelings in charge, you will end up eating what feels good and kills slowly. You'll wind up like a huge whale with a ticking time bomb in it.

While we always have it at the back of our minds to eat healthy, stay hydrated, and sleep well, all this is often easier said than done. It's like a very vivid dream you have and then forget when you wake up. Keep in mind the keyword here is will. Will! As in the driving need to fulfill a set goal. *Not will, as in Will.I.Am.*

Psychology and Emotional Eating

You might wonder what psychology has to do with emotional eating. Well, psychology studies human behavior. It studies why humans act the way they do. For people trying to find a way to manage emotional eating, psychology will help. How?

- *It addresses your character.* Your eating behaviours and patterns would need to be observed so an action plan *tailored to your needs* can be designed.
- *You can identify your thought patterns.* Your thoughts and emotions would need to be analyzed. You can then discover what your emotional triggers are. Once your cognitive pattern has been

thoroughly explored with the help of a licensed professional, they can then figure out a fitting solution to the problem.

The Road Ahead

The truth is no matter what solutions are proffered; they just won't work unless you're ready to make a change. You have to be willing to drop emotional eating and lead a healthier life. Your decision must be unwavering. This requires putting a lot of effort into achieving success, limiting distractions, and setting targets.

You also have to be self-aware. Become mindful. Do not act unconsciously. Just observe and watch for triggers that induce specific cravings. Then, be careful of what you eat and how much you do it.

Try replacing your sugary confections with something sugary, but healthy. Like an apple, or pineapple. Whenever you start to have your cravings for a pastry, try to replace is with something healthier. It won't be easy, but where there's a will, there's a way. How do you get the will? Find your why. When you have solid, concrete reasons for wanting to make a change, you'll find the "how" gets that much more achievable.

There is nothing more satisfying than looking back at some mistakes you have made and seeing that you have overcome them. Yes, the past may have shaped your undesirable present. But the present shapes the future, Every moment you spend wallowing in self-pity, body shaming yourself, and languishing in the throes of a broken heart, just keeps you from achieving the final goal.

If you stick with me, I'm going to give you the tools you need to overcome your emotional eating. You just have to decide that you can, and you will. Against all odds. It's no secret people tend to get what they want if they put their all into it.

So are you with me? I want you all in. I want you to remember why you started, whenever you want to quit. I want you to know I'm rooting for you. I want you to know I've seen countless people beat emotional eating. I've seen it happen, so I know it can be done. I know *you can do it.* But I can only hold your hand. You're going to have to put one foot in front of the other and take this journey with me. Can you do it? Will you do it?

Are you worth it?

Don't turn the page until you realize and feel deeply in your bones the only correct answer to that question.

Yes. You are worth it. So very worth it.

Chapter 3: How Do You Compare?

Before I go any further, I want to make sure you know the difference between overeating here and there and an eating disorder, which is a medical issue. One of the reasons why I want to take time to look into this a bit more in depth is because I don't want any of you to worry about if you have a full-blown eating disorder where you need to find help to overcome it or if you just overeat from time to time and all you need to do is watch your portions better. Another reason is because overeating stems into other eating disorders, such as anorexia and bulimia. In a nutshell, I want you to know where you sit on the line before you head one direction or the other.

Overeating

Earlier, we discussed how overeating is simply eating more than your body's daily calorie intake. This means people usually consume way more than they should during holidays, family gathers, social outings, and other special times. If it's not during one of these special meals, they won't generally overeat as they control their portions better. But this doesn't mean that when people aren't eating at these special meals, they won't overeat. In fact, most people don't even realize they are overeating.

We're millennials so we live in a fast-paced world. For most of us, our days typically consist of getting up and getting ready to go to work or school. From there, we go from class to class, or we work throughout our day. We then run errands, go to another job, go to an internship, and then get home. If we have children, we also make sure they get to school, day care, or their activities. When we live in such a fast-paced world, we don't always get the time to eat. And, sometimes, when we do, we need to eat so fast so we don't miss our next errand, class, task, or anything else we need to do.

The problem with this is when we eat so fast, we're not able to pay attention to the cue of fullness from our body nor can our stomach and brain keep up with how fast we are eating. Therefore, like I've touched on before, by the time we feel our sense of fullness, we've already overeaten. Just take for a moment and think about how often you eat on the run or quickly in order to get to the next thing you need to do.

Another point to this about is how often do you skip a meal because you're too busy or you don't have enough money to buy something when you have left your lunch at home. If you take a moment to think about this, it probably happens more than you realized, especially if you're a college student, working full-time with a family, or both. The problem is, this can also cause overeating. When we skip meals, we tend to feel like we're hungry than we actually are the next time we have a meal. Because of this, we will overeat as we eat too fast, or we grab more than necessary because we feel like we have to finish the food. When our eyes are bigger than our stomachs, which often happens when we skip a meal, we tend to overeat. In order to avoid this, all you really need to do is make sure you don't skip that meal. As a millennial myself, I know that this can be tough because we are so busy; however, it's extremely important to remember because overeating leads to more serious eating disorders.

Another way we overeat and don't realize it is by keeping ourselves distracted as we eat. For example, how often do you sit in front of the television screen, phone, or another device to catch up on Facebook, Twitter, or some other social media platform when you're having a bite to eat? Maybe you do other things like homework, tasks at work, or just chill on your phone and catch up with your friends. All of these types of actions can cause overeating due to one main reason. We're not paying attention to how much we're eating, and unless we portioned our food, this means we can easily overeat. This is called mindless eating, which means you continue to eat without thinking about it or paying attention to your body's cues that you're full.

Now I want you to think about some of the reasons that cause overeating and notice how often you take part in these activities. If you realize it's a weekly activity and typically two or more times a week, you're on the path to becoming a binge eater. If you notice that you don't do this very often but often enough and it's become a personal concern, you're an overeater, and there are a lot of ways you can change this behavior before you become a binge eater.

The biggest way to make sure you don't overeat is to pay attention. Not only do you want to pay attention to how much you're eating, but you also want to pay attention to how much food you're putting on your plate. One of the best things to do is to portion your food. This will help you stay on track with the right amount of food you should be consuming. Another tip is to stay away from devices when you eat. The best thing to do is to sit down at a kitchen table and focus on eating. You also can help yourself be chewing your food slowly.

Symptoms of Binge Eating Disorder

Now that you better understand what overeating is and what causes it, let's look more closely into the symptoms of an eating disorder. After we discuss this, it should help you better realize the details between a full-blown eating disorder and overeating enough where you know which path you need to head down so you can overcome overeating or binge eating.

There are many symptoms for you to pay attention to so you can see if you have a binge eating disorder or not. One of the symptoms is you binge regularly, which means at least twice a week for a period of six months. Another symptom of binge eating is you take in a large amount of food in a short period of time. When I say a short period of time, I'm not talking about twenty minutes or a half hour. I'm talking about a period of two hours. This is one of the biggest ways you realize if you binge eat or overeat. When you overeat, you usually only do so for a few minutes. But when you binge eat, you will continue to eat whatever you can for a couple of hours. When you are in the middle of a binge eating episode, you literally feel like you can't stop, so you keep on eating.

Other symptoms of binge eating disorder are eating when you're full, grabbing something to eat even when you don't feel hungry, and eating by yourself because it's too embarrassing to eat with other people. All these symptoms are signs of binge eating and signs that you should begin to work on taking more control of you're eating before it's too late.

But these aren't the only symptoms to pay attention to if you think you might be a binge eater. Another symptom is to pay attention to how you feel and act after a binge eating episode. For example, binge eaters often feel guilty about all the food they just ate. They also feel depressed, anxious, worthless, or disgusted by their actions afterward. These emotions will also bring you into a cycle with binge eating because they will make you feel so bad that you will turn to food in order to comfort yourself.

Chapter 4: At War With Food?

War has been declared. Swords have been drawn. *Time to battle!*

You might be wondering how you can be at war with food. We're going to get into that right now. See, as an emotional eater, there is constant war between your will and your cravings. Every single time you saw the cravings win and you were helpless to stop it? Those were squabbles compared to what is coming.

Laying Siege!

A war has been declared and you are going to have to be your own knight in shining armor because this is a battle that mercenaries can't fight on your behalf. Every failed attempt you have had with dealing with your emotional eating has brought you closer to this moment of decision.

When your emotions start to get frayed as a response to negative stimuli, you can take measures to control your cravings. More often than not, you will indulge in emotional eating when you are at your weakest emotionally.

Go Do Something ELSE!

I don't care what it is, as long as it's not eating, and it's not going to kill you. Listen to some music. Listen to a TED Talk or some podcast or something. Talk to some friends. Go out. Go jog. Cycle. Do anything *but* eat at that moment.

Here's why.

Hunger and Cravings Come In Waves

If you've always just given in to all your cravings, chances are you've never noticed hunger actually comes in waves. It's not something that hits you full on and just keeps getting worse until you finally shove something into your piehole.

Are You In Denial?

One of the hardest things ever is fixing the results caused by a problem you created. If you're going to beat this thing, then the first step is acknowledging you actually have a problem.

Some people do not believe they have a problem. Especially when they believe they are eating "well." This happens when they rationalize it with various thoughts, like wanting to have a fuller figure, or to fill out their cheeks so they're no longer sunken. But then what happens when they successfully achieve those goals? *They just. Won't. Stop. Eating!* It won't be a pretty sight once your behind gets more *generous.*

If you've read up to this point and you're still trying to suss out whether or not you actually have a food problem, be honest with yourself. This is why it is a war. A battle of wills. Head versus stomach. Only the strongest man wins. You could always try weighing your options , but you don't have many. If you don't work now to stop your emotional eating habits, your self-esteem will be thrown into the mud and trod upon like so much *nothing*.

Fall In Love With Food

Wait… What? Yes, I said that. If you're at war with food, then that needs to end NOW. It's not food you need to be at war with. It's your own emotions. It's all the temptations which call to you, asking you to eat one more cookie, one more slice, one more fork full.

How do you fix this? *Love food that treats you good.* Imagine you're in a relationship with someone, and no matter how much you love them, they always make you feel like such utter crap. What do you do then? Of COURSE you ditch them!

So why are you still in a love affair with foods that treat you like shit? Yes, I cussed. I did that to snap you out of it. You know you feel like crap when you eat them. So fall in love with the good stuff instead! This way, you get rid of the guilt that keeps you trapped in the cycle of emotional eating. I'm not asking you to go on a diet. I'm asking you to fall in love with food worth loving. I'm asking you to love your body and treat it better. It's not going to be easy, but you can lean on friends and family. You can seek out professional help. I know you'll pull through!

Temptations

The main factor in emotional eating is the presence of temptation. If you know there is anything that might cause you to relapse into old habits, remove it. If it seems too much for you then flee!

There is no cowardice in retreat. You go to fight another day, bolder and stronger. I don't care if people laugh at you because of how fast you bolt out the room when someone walks in with a box of pizza. Do whatever you have to. Slowly and steadily you will win the battle.

Restrictive Dieting and Emotional Eating

For a lot of people, emotional eating is just a part of a wheel or a cycle formed from restrictive dieting. You see, people are of the very wrong impression that it is only people who do not eat a lot when they are hungry that become emotional eaters. This misconception is why a lot of people are caught up in this vicious cycle. First they eat. Then they feel guilty for eating. To deal with the shame, they eat again. Wash, rinse, and repeat.

This is a cycle that has to be broken! It is a cycle of shame and self-derision!
Is it just me, or is it the food?

Over the years, food addiction has become a topic of interest among scientists. These scientists have come up with theories that state that foods rich in sugar, fat and salt are addictive, and they act upon the brain like some hard drugs such as cocaine!

The crazy thing is, the normal treatment for addiction is withdrawal and abstinence. That sure can't happen with food because we need it to survive.

Other researchers have asserted it may not be the food that is addictive, but it's more likely the individual who is prone to addiction. They propose it's the continuous cycle of shame and indulgence that creates addictive dependence, not the food itself.

If your emotional eating has progressed to a full blown addiction to food, then you have to try as much as possible not to bring your comfort food to your comfort zone. If you do, that's asking for trouble! One can't be too careful. The fact you are not a coward doesn't mean you should test your will unnecessarily.

Let's be real for a second here. You wouldn't leave a pyromaniac around a box of matches and some gasoline, would you? Then why would you allow all sorts of foods you *know* you're helplessly addicted to when you're trying to beat this thing?

Exactly.

Chapter 5: What Kind of Eater Are You?

What kind of foods are you often found eating? Your daily eating pattern can determine what kind of eater you are.

Are you usually found eating pork roast at dinner, or a bowl of fresh veggies? Are you more of a Mac and cheese person? All these speak volumes about the kind of eater you are if you are not yet aware of it.

Are your foods almost always paper wrapped from a fast food joint? Do you almost always eat while watching the games, chick flick or a horror movie? Have you always seen your self-accepting free food? Have you ever found yourself eating even when there is no gnawing hunger in your belly?

If you fit any of the descriptions given above, then you have most likely developed an unhealthy eating habit or pattern. Habits that will eventually sabotage every weight loss program you might have.

A lot of times, it is very simple to identify bad eating habits. Like when food becomes the only solution to your problems, or when it becomes the only stress relief method you can think of. When you start to think it is impossible that anything but food could make you better at that point. Sometimes, these signs are not clear enough so a person can go for a long time in ignorant bliss. Sometimes these habits become so much a part of you, you do not even realise you are doing them. They become unconscious actions. Dictated by your cravings and not your mind.

There are various types of eating habits and they vary from person to person. Experts have asserted these patterns are determined mostly by a person's behavior. With the majority of affected people being overweight or obese.

Stress Eating

You may notice you eat a bit more when you are stressed, but you won't always associate it with emotional eating. Especially when you are always munching on small things, which add up to become bigger things by the end of your day at work or school.

Some people are always in a panic about what to eat and how to eat it. Most times because they find it difficult making a choice, they end up at the local restaurant, eating something oily and salty. This develops into a very unhealthy lifestyle. Because as is human nature, we always go for the simplest option in a time of confusion.

Task Eating

The type of eating pattern people are less likely to discover they have is *task eating*. People who always work easier with a bit of something in their mouths. Maybe a bit of chocolate while doing the laundry, some chips while cooking, a bit of gum while writing or even some soda while reading. People don't tend to notice this habit because the mind is occupied with the more important and difficult of the two tasks, the other just being the dormant of the two activities.

Multitasking!

Sometimes, people also eat because they're lonely. If this is you, you eat when you're alone. You eat to fill the void inside. That's really the only reason you're reaching for that 5th slice of pizza, even though your gut started to protest at slice 3.

This is not just some made up thing. Research shows there is a high likelihood for binge eaters to always feel lonely. This lonely eater has more fat than the rest of society, and tends to each at very odd, irregular times. Did you know loneliness actually stresses you out? Go figure!

Excuses, and How to Beat Them

We all know fast foods are known for their high fat and sugar or salt content, yet some people would rather eat fast food than eat healthy.

After all it's fast!
They do not want to sacrifice the time needed to buy some of the groceries and then to cook. Some give the excuse they do not know how to cook and yet there are healthier food options out there.

You have to keep note of your eating habits, so as to make it easier to find a solution to help yourself. Once you have discovered that the flesh is weak, but the mind is willing, you have to put measures to ensure you do not fall back into temptation.

Okay Aron, What Do I DO?

- Clear out that stash of chips you have in your cabinet.

- Buy some veggies and low calorie foods to store in your fridge, so you do not have a reason to drive out to that grocery store.

- If munching on something crunchy helps soothe you or relax you, try a healthy alternative like carrots! They're just as crunchy as chips, and so much better for you.

So, why did you just make that face?

"But Aron! It's not the same thing! It's not *my* thing!" Well do you want to be healthy or not? Then you have to learn to fall in love with the good stuff! Being and staying healthy should be *everybody's* thing!

Feeling Discouraged?

Now, you're probably thinking this is not worth the time and effort you're going to have to put in. But when people say, "This is not worth it," what they're really saying is I am not worth it. So I'm going to ask you again, are you, or are you not worth good health? Do you deserve it or not?

I said you are not just going to quit right off the bat. I already mentioned there is no off switch. So what's going to happen is you are going to wean yourself of these comfort foods. Since it's like a fix, quitting abruptly will do more harm than good.

You feel tired already? I know.

You will have to take it slowly. One step at a time. We will talk about how to do just that in the coming chapters. You just have to know you are not alone! You picked up this book for a reason. You picked it up because you know something's wrong. You've read this far because you're desperate for change. You'll get that change, but you're going to have to put in the work, amigo.

Chapter 6: Energy Your Body Needs

What we believe about food and how we perceive food plays an integral part in our eating habits and our lives in general. Although more and more people are becoming health conscious and they have a positive perception of food, there are just as many people who have a negative impression of food.

Some people view food as the enemy and regard most food types as either bad in some way or just plain fattening. They consider most food to hurt their body in some or other way. They therefore either eat extremely little or they tend to have extremely unhealthy eating habits.

This is also one of the significant causes of guilt, associated with food. Many people tend to experience feelings of guilt even before they eat something. The reality is that it is not the food that is fattening, it is the negative emotion, the sin which is associated with it.

Our emotions affect so many aspects of our lives, not only our eating habits but our lives as a whole. Thus, when negative emotions are "attached" to food, food then becomes the enemy. How can one then enjoy a meal, if you are already thinking of all the negative aspects of it?

This is one of the most important things which needs to change, to be able to eat mindfully. The words "guilt" and "food" do not belong in the same sentence. Food should be viewed as neutral and as sustenance. Just as a vehicle needs fuel, so do our bodies need food.

Mindful eating is not something new or practice which has recently been developed or invented by someone. Many people have been practicing conscious consumption for decades.

Eating mindfully means to be aware of your thoughts, your feelings, your emotions and your reason for eating. It is about enjoying your food, savoring the flavor, paying attention to what the food looks like, the aroma and how it makes you feel. It is about being fully aware of every moment and every mouthful and the experience you have while eating.

This should be a moment of quiet bliss for the soul and your meal being sustenance to the body.

Many people do not eat mindfully at all, for a variety of reasons. But, what can we do to assist us in eating mindfully? One obvious answer would be to practice awareness. Awareness of self, knowledge of the food you are about to eat, awareness of your surroundings and understanding of how the food makes you feel. additional perk to mindful eating.

When we are eating mindfully, we want to find foods that are good for our soul as these will be good for our mind and body, and we want to stay away from foods that our mindless stomach tells us it wants.

Importance of Food

If your life is busy, you might find that it is much faster and convenient to turn to finger foods or comfort foods than it is to take the time to eat something that might sustain you longer. Although it takes a little extra time, the benefits of choosing foods that sustain you longer are invaluable. The extra time spent choosing or preparing these foods will be worth the time spent on the process.

Nutritious Foods Sustain Longer. When a food sustains you longer, you go longer without being fixated on what you are going to eat next. Cravings are reduced, and you will find that you feel great. Mindful eaters look for opportunities to choose foods that best serve their bodies and overall well being.

There are a variety of foods that will keep you full longer. Popcorn, eggs, vegetables, cottage cheese, and healthy fats such as almonds, walnuts, and pistachio nuts are some that will keep you from feeling hungry so quickly after a meal. As with other types of food, there is enough of a variety to keep you from feeling limited in your choices.

One step in the mindful eating process is learning to choose nutritious foods. There is nothing wrong with having occasional sweet treats, or other non-nutritious treats. It becomes a problem when people believe they must have treats at every meal. Choosing nutritious food is to choose those foods that will keep you from becoming hungry again too quickly. Some foods might be pleasing to the taste buds, but they leave you feeling dissatisfied. While examining the different food groups, it is important to note that people need foods from all groups. Balance is the key.

Vegetables

When it comes to mindful eating, vegetables are often the first category of food people focus on. This is usually because, when we discuss healthy eating, people automatically think of vegetables. They are definitely on the list of foods to eat when you're mindfully eating; for example, making sure there are more vegetables on your plate than starch and fatty food.

Fruit

Real fresh fruit is some of the best fruit to pick when you're working on mindful eating habits. While canned fruit can be good for a snack, you want to watch what type of canned fruit you get because these can often be high in sugar and corn syrup, which isn't good for you.

Vitamins

Many people are disregarding the true potential that vitamins have. They think that vitamins are simple molecules which are important for sustaining life, but the reality is that vitamins can do much more than that. If you ask me vitamins have the power to change our lives and appearance.

Vitamins can help us lose weight, gain bone and muscle strength and improve immune function. There are many professional athletes who use vitamin supplements to increase protein synthesis and endurance. Some scientists believe that ultra high doses can even cure deadly virus and bacterial infections. You probably heard about many health benefits, but what are vitamins in essence?

Vitamins are tiny organic molecules which are required in small amount for various processes throughout the body. Their main role is to speed up and enhance chemical reactions that create bone, muscle and skin. It is important to get daily recommended amounts of vitamins to prevent weakness and serious diseases.

Usually, we obtain vitamins from food, but we can also generate vitamins in our body. For example, vitamin D is generated when we expose our skin to sunlight.

Vitamins are divided into two categories: water-soluble and fat-soluble vitamins. Water-soluble vitamins easily dissolve in water and like water they need to be replenished daily. Fat-soluble vitamins dissolve in fat and are stored in the liver and other organs. They do not need to be replenished every day.

Do not use vitamin supplements and pills, because high doses can lead to toxicity. Vitamin toxicity can cause many serious problems including nerve damage.

Consult your doctor if you think you are not obtaining enough vitamins.

The best sources are fruits and vegetables. It is found in colored fruits such as grapefruit and cantaloupe. Vegetables, such as potatoes, carrots, pumpkin and broccoli are great sources. It comes from animal sources also such as fish oils, meat, liver and kidneys.

The good thing is that vitamins are found in many fruits and vegetables. Basically, there is no fruit or vegetable that does not contain at least a trace of this vitamin. Fruits with highest content are citrus fruits, kiwi, guava, strawberries, cranberries, blueberries, raspberries, mango and pineapple. Vegetables with highest content are cabbage, spinach, potato, tomato, broccoli and winter squash.

Whole Grains

Whole grain foods are very important in your diet and, while, like all foods, you need to be mindful about how much you eat, they do make the foods to eat list. There are many health benefits to whole grain foods, such as they are high in fiber. If you suffer from things like constipation, which can happen with poor eating habits, these foods will help regulate your system, which will help in digestion, and make you feel better overall. There are a lot of options of breads out there, and regular white and wheat breads are not the healthiest. Instead, you want to find whole grain breads as these will be healthier than any other bread. While they are a bit more expensive, you will be able to notice a difference in your mind, body, and soul.

Dairy

Like any other food group, dairy should not be overdone, but you do need to have a sufficient amount of it. Dairy products are linked to bone health. Vitamin D provides calcium and phosphorus. Potassium is also provided by certain dairy products. There is protein in some dairy products so you can get protein and dairy in one food choice.

Dairy foods such as milk, cheese, butter, yogurt, cottage cheese provide nutrients you need. Some breakfast cereals are rich in these nutrients. There is enough of a variety that you should be able to choose something you enjoy.

Sugar

As with all other food ingredients, moderation is the key. Often, human beings have a difficult time practicing moderation. More always seems better, but that is not always the case. Mindfulness puts the idea of "more" into perspective. With mindful eating, you realize that you can have a moderate amount of most food types. There are times when you do not need them, then, there are times when a little is acceptable.

Many nutritionists believe that white refined sugar is the source of health problems. In some cases, that is true. In other cases, going to extremes to eliminate sugar from one's diet can cause more stress than it relieves. Some experts recommend substituting honey for white sugar. Once again, whatever your source of sweetener, moderation is the key to healthy eating.

A great deal of controversy has been present over artificial sweeteners. Many people use them in their tea, coffee, or other drinks because they believe they do not need the extra calories of a natural sweetener. Of course, diabetics often turn to this source because of their own health issues.

Carbohydrates

Carbohydrates do not come without a bit of controversy, particularly in the health world. There are health experts who believe you should limit your carb intake. The South Beach Diet and the Atkins Diet have been popular as well as convincing. According to these diet programs, limiting your carb intake will turn your body into a fat burning machine. The problem is that carbs are needed for energy.

As with any other food product, moderation is key. Once again, mindful eating comes in with assessing how certain foods make you feel after you have eaten them. If a particular food drains you of energy, you might need to eat less of it. If you feel great after eating a certain type of food, you know that it has just what your body needs.

Chapter 7: Cravings and Temptations

Temptations

We all battle with temptations not only people with binge disorder. Then again, it is easier for most people to simply say no and let the temptation go, but people with binge disorder find it almost impossible.

What is it that has you by the throat? Is it the smell of fresh baked goods, ice-cream, chocolate, donuts or crisps and cookies? Take the foods that you love most to binge on, and remove them all from your home and office. Clear out your fridge, clean out the cupboards and re-stock with healthy alternatives.

Removing temptations from your reach is easier than resisting them. Replace your favorite food, or snack with a healthier alternative.

Here are some suggestions:

- *Sugar can be replaced with honey. If feeling like something sweet rather eat a fruit or two, instead of sweets.*
- *Chocolates can be replaced with nuts, or healthy cereal.*

- *Salty snacks, such as crisps can be replaced by a handful of salted peanuts.*
- *Fried and oily foods can be replaced by a variety of cheeses, tuna on a cracker, or even some boiled eggs with spice.*

Find healthy alternatives to your temptations, and nip them in the butt.

Cravings

Don't keep any unhealthy snacks at your home or the office. Cravings, are one of the problems experienced by people that have binge eating disorder.

Stock your fridge, and cupboards with an assortment of healthy foods. This way when watching a movie or reading a book in bed, and you have a craving for cake or crisps, you may alternatively just eat an apple, or have a fruit smoothie, as it is easier accessible. Most people will not go through the trouble of getting dressed, and going to the shop to buy other foods, if they have something available.

The secret to preventing cravings from taking over, is to remove temptations from your home and office.

Chapter 8: Respect Your Body

Acknowledge your hereditary outline. Similarly as an individual with a shoe size of eight would not expect sensibly to crush into a size six, it is similarly useless (and awkward) to have a comparable desire about body size. Regard your body so you can feel good about what your identity is. It's difficult to dismiss the diet attitude in the event that you are ridiculous and excessively incredulous of your body shape.

Body carefulness sires body stress, which generates nourishment stress, which energizes the cycle of dieting. So what do you do, simply overlook it? Creep into a dull cavern, escape the world and eat everything in sight? No. In any case for whatever length of time that you are at war with your body it will be hard to be at harmony with yourself and nourishment. With each slandering look in the reflection, the Food Police addition control, and with that comes pledges of just one more diet.

Has all the self-hatred due to your body made a difference? Has abiding on your flawed body parts helped you to progress toward becoming more slender, or only exacerbated you feel? Does berating yourself each time you step on the scale make your weight any less? We still can't seem to discover one customer who says that concentrating on their body in such negative manners is useful.

Studies have demonstrated that the more you center on your body, the more terrible you feel about yourself. However the body torment game goes on—Mirror, reflect on the divider, who's the slimmest of all?

It's difficult to get away from the body torment game when the entire nation is playing it. For the sake of wellness, a lean and hard shape has turned into the body symbol since the nineties. Self-broadcasted wellness masters demand that you can "shape" your body as though it were a chunk of earth, that you can change your hereditary shape with an oxygen consuming episode and puff.

We are enthusiastic backers of being fit and perceive the medical advantages of activity, yet we believe we should bring up that unreasonable desires are being painted.

It is broadly acknowledged in the exploration network that you can't spot lose fat in only one determined spot). So how might it be that you will shape your body by chipping away at certain body parts? Indeed, you can fabricate explicit muscles through quality and obstruction preparing. Furthermore, truly, you can lose generally muscle to fat ratio through oxygen consuming activity. In any case, you can't by and by select where that fat will be lost. It's conceivable to manufacture muscle underneath fat layers, yet this isn't the idea of body chiseling that most overweight individuals have at the top of the priority list.

The most effective method to Respect Your Body

Consider regarding your body in two different ways: first, by making it agreeable, what's more, second, by gathering its essential needs. You have the right to be agreeable.

You have the right to get your essential needs met. Or on the other hand the more hopeless you feel, the more hopeless you'll be.

Think about these fundamental premises of body regard:

• My body has the right to be encouraged.

• My body has the right to be treated with respect.

• My body has the right to be dressed easily and in the way I am acquainted with.

• My body has the right to be contacted lovingly and with regard.

• My body has the right to move easily.

Chapter 9: The Pressures of Being a Millennial

The age range for a millennial in 2019 is from 23 to 38—anyone born between the years of 1981–1996. It's this age group that's often facing the pressures of graduating from college, starting a career, beginning a family, and working toward building a life. While every age group faces their own daily struggles, millennials tend to face a set of different struggles than other age groups. Because of their struggles, millennials try to find ways they can cope with their struggles, stress, and emotions. For many others, including myself, the coping mechanism became binge eating.

For me, binge eating was a way that not only made me feel in better control of my life but also a place for my emotions to hide. Like most others who suffer from binge eating, I didn't see anything wrong with it at first. Food helped me ease my stress for a period of time. However, as I kept eating more and more, I started to realize that what I was doing wasn't healthy. Of course, this didn't help my emotions as I began to feel more overwhelmed, but it also didn't stop me from continuing to binge eat.

I also started to feel alone in my struggle. I felt embarrassed, angry, and sad about what I had done to myself. To find out that I was actually out of control with my eating instead of in control became devastating. The feeling of isolation began to take hold of me as I continued to struggle within myself. How could I tell anyone that I turned myself into a binge eater? I didn't want my friends and family to judge me. I wanted to make this point about feeling alone because now I know that I never was alone. Not only are there millions of other people who struggle with binge eating, but if I would have reached out to my friends and family, they wouldn't have judged me or left me alone to deal with my binge eating struggle.

I truly believe that one of the best ways to start helping yourself if you're struggling with binge eating is to know that you are not alone. There are millions of people who are going through the same struggle right now. Not only will you be able to find support through your friends and family, but there are tons of eating disorder groups which can give you the support you need to help beat this battle. I really can't stress this point enough. In fact, I want you to read the following words out loud, "I am not alone." Now I want you to repeat them as many times as you need to so you can begin to truly believe that you are not alone.

It's a Daily Struggle

The struggle of dealing with an eating disorder is a daily one. Even when I did my best during the day to not binge eat, it was still a struggle. In reality, binge eating and any other eating disorder are like any addition in the books. Just because you don't do it one day doesn't mean you're cured, it's not that bad, or that you didn't think about eating more. Most days, it's a struggle from the time you get up until the time you go to bed. The want of needing more food is almost constantly in the back of your mind.

If you get frustrated, angry, sad, or tired because you feel this struggle is too much to handle, you're not alone. Nearly everyone who deals with binge eating feels the same way. It seems that some type of food is always near our fingertips, and in those moments we have a strong enough willpower to say no, it feels like it takes every ounce of your willpower to not pick up that piece of food. This makes us tired and then, and in those moments we give in, it makes us feel defeated.

All these emotions are completely normal. It's estimated that over 2 million people in the United States suffer from binge eating disorder, which means there are around 2 million people who have dealt with the same struggle with binge eating disorder as you do. For them, it's also a daily struggle.

Even though millennials are known to have more struggles than previous generations, they are also very tough and determined, which makes them easily overcome these struggles. Even when we deal with bumps in the road, such as eating disorders, we band together and are able to overcome them.

Stereotypes

One of the biggest things millennials deal with are stereotypes that other generations, and some millennials, have. Most of these stereotypes focus on the negative characteristics, such as we're self-absorbed, lazy, and obsessed with technology. For many people, stereotypes can put a damper on their mood, and if they are constantly reminded of the stereotypes, which most millennials are, it's harder to reach the point where you don't see yourself of a stereotype.

With this said, I want you to remember one thing. You are not the stereotypes. You're not the stereotypes people have given millennials, and you're not the stereotypes attached to people who suffer from eating disorders. You are bigger and better than the stereotype. People always say, "To prove stereotypes wrong, you need to do the opposite and prove them wrong to people." While this is a great advice, the only thing you need to focus on right now is proving you to yourself. You need to show yourself that you can and will accomplish anything because you're a millennial.

Chapter 10: Stress Eating

Stress Management

Life is not easy, and no-one ever said it would be, as we are constantly facing a variety of situations daily, from a very young age. We learn that life's ups and downs aren't something to be controlled. It is however, something that we can learn to live with, learn to handle and cope with.

Stress has numerous effects on the human body, and it can cause a variation of health problems. Binge eating is only one of the problems stress brings on, but there is also heart disease, cholesterol problems and many more.

Learning to cope with stress, or how to manage it will help you immensely, not only will you be able to control binge eating, but furthermore you will be able to live a healthy life.

Not all of our daily, weekly or monthly stresses can be avoided, thus we need to find ways to manage, without excessive eating. There are various ways of resolving stressful situations, whether it is through breathing exercises, relaxation strategies or even meditation. The aim is to find something that helps you to relax, eliminating the stress factors from your life.

Manage Stress the Healthy Way

Why do you have stress? This is important to consider, as the cause of your stress firstly needs to be addressed, and only then can it be managed. Is it your bills, family responsibilities, career pressure, or do you simply not have enough hours within one day to do all that needs doing? You may feel overwhelmed, but in fact you have control! You must stand up and take back your life! Take control of your mind and thoughts, your schedule, besides your emotions. Find ways that helps you to cope, and work through the stresses in your life. Binge eating may soothe you in the moment, yet there are healthier alternatives available.

Try one, or all of the following to alleviate your stress:

- *Set limits – Learn to say 'NO' to people. If you do not want to do something, or really don't have the time, just say 'NO'. Don't place yourself under more pressure. You can only do so much!*
- *Exercises – Whether you jog, ride a bicycle, dance or just go for walks, do it at least three*

times a week. Regular exercise is proven to aid in reducing stress, plus as a bonus, it is also a great way to keep your body healthy.

- *Hot Topics – Does certain discussions boil your blood? So, why talk about them at all? Simply cross these topics off your list. You can tell family and friends, that you would prefer not to talk about these, and if you find yourself in a discussion socially that could raise your stress levels, just walk away.*

- *Distractions – We are blessed to be living in a digital age, use these to your own benefit. Listen to music, play audio books, or even games on your tablet or phone. Distract your mind when you feel stressed.*

- *Re-schedule – Sit down and have a look at your daily activities, are there to many things to do, and too little time? Scale down, re-schedule and priorities. Make a list of things that just 'have' to be done, and things that 'should' be done. Things that don't fit either group can be discarded immediately, then prioritize the rest.*

- *Activities – Find activities you enjoy doing, whether alone or in a group. These can be things like painting, singing, pottery or crafts. Find something to keep your hands and mind busy, this is a proven method of stress relief.*

- *Environment – Remove yourself from places that makes you uncomfortable. If traffic is an issue, find a quieter route home. If the news is upsetting, just don't watch it. You can do shopping online, thus staying away from shopping centers, if they make you uncomfortable.*

Chapter 11: Health and Nutrition

Healthy Meals and Snacks

Excessive and unhealthy eating is one of the main problem with binge disorder. It holds multiple health risks, except for the emotional scaring it causes. People who eat unhealthy foods, in large amounts, over long periods of time, are opening themselves up to other diseases such as cancer, diabetes, heart disease and more. Your body needs protein, minerals, vitamins and small amounts of sugars, carbohydrates and more. Over dosing your body on just one, or two of these can lead to bigger problems.

You need to eat a minimum of three meals per day. It is also recommended to eat two healthy snacks per day. One between breakfast and lunch, and the other between lunch and supper. People with binge disorder must set up a schedule for themselves, and keep to it!

Start your day with a healthy breakfast. Include a fruit or two, some yoghurt, healthy cereals, or a vegetable smoothie. This meal must be filling and nutritious. Do not skip any of your meals during the day, and keep strictly to the times of each meal you have set for yourself!

For snacks you can eat fruit, vegetable sticks or have smoothies. It must be easy to prepare, quick and not overfilling. Keep it light and healthy. Once again, same time every day!

Dinner meals must include some protein, (fish, chicken, lean beef), lots of green vegetables, and only one starch such as, potatoes, rice and macaroni. Try to stay clear of breads, cakes and foods that are processed.

Eating regularly and healthy will aid you in eating less. Fresh fruit and vegetables are also the best option, as they contain more high-nutrients, which provides a fuller feeling, and keeps the body going longer periods.

Nutrients

Eating less may not always be the easiest feat to overcome. Yet, if you replace the unhealthy foods you consume with healthy alternatives, it does make a difference, especially in the long run.

Studies have shown that most people consume less than 60% of the suggested intake of fruits, vegetables, fish, dairy and whole grain products. These are ideal to incorporate into your schedule as snacks, increasing your nutrient intake daily.

Healthy snacks also aid in sustaining your sugar levels throughout the day. This is important to maintain, as low sugar levels will leave you feeling tired. Snacks with high sugar levels will only help in causing extreme highs and lows, leaving you with an ultimate energy drain. Try carrot sticks, cabbage salad, cucumbers or other vegetables with a dip to sustain energy levels throughout the day.

Eat food in small portions, as even healthy foods can add to your weight if consumed in excessive amounts. Have healthy snacks on hand if hunger should come walking in, then you know, you are prepared. Nonetheless, if you keep to balanced meals and a strict schedule, all should be just fine.

Eating healthier will leave you feeling happier, less stressed and even more productive. You will also have a fuller, longer life and age with elegance.

Get into a habit of eating slower, savor each bite, focus on chewing. You can even count your bites, if you need to, or chew each one no less than ten times.

Chapter 12: Behind the Scenes of the Food Industry

In this chapter, we will learn all about the different ingredients that big corporations use to make their processed food as addictive as possible, causing consumers to want them more and more. These highly addictive components can be found in fast food, junk food, convenience store items, and so much more. Together, we will take a closer and more in-depth look behind the scenes at how these trick our brain into binge eating without us even knowing it.

How Big Corporations are Manipulating Chemicals in Food to Get Consumers Addicted

Have you ever wondered why once you pop a piece of fries into your mouth, you just can't bring yourself to stop? Or when you indulge in a spoonful of delectable ice cream goodness, you find yourself emptying out the whole tub in just a matter of minutes? Binge Eating Disorder is a serious condition that involves both the emotional and mental aspect of a person's well-being, but external forces are also at play. When it comes to making junk food as irresistible as possible, big conglomerates and multinational companies may also be at fault. Not only are commercials and persistent ads to blame for all of the temptations, but the manufacturers of food themselves manipulate the ingredients that they use in order to get consumers utterly hooked to their product.

For instance, fast food is incredibly addictive because of all the heaps and heaps of sugar, salt, and fat packed into every meal. In the form of hydrogenated and partially hydrogenated oils and high fructose corn syrup, these seemingly harmless everyday kitchen ingredients can become the sole culprits to unhealthy weight gain and bad cholesterol. With every serving, fat and salt levels will likely be way too high, and will ultimately exceed your body's regular needs. As a result, these trigger substances spike up your addition to the junk food, keeping you coming back for more and more.

The tricky thing is that our brain actually thinks these foods are rewards. The food affects our brains and how we make decisions, and because we can get these "rewarding" foods at a very affordable cost, the decision to buy and consume them becomes, well, a no-brainer. Add that to the fact that heading down to your nearest fast food joint for a quick fat fix (or even having the food delivered right to your doorstep with no effort at all) is as convenient as ever, and you've got yourself a foolproof recipe for making really, really bad food decisions.

Also pushing you to give in to the temptation (and therefore disrupting your impulse control) are flavoring agents like MSG. Monosodium Glutamate (MSG) is added to food as a form of concentrated salt to enhance flavors. It's cheap, readily available, and even "generally recognized as safe" by the Food and Drug Administration. But even so, it can suppress your appetite, causing you to feel like you still want more even if you are already full. It has also been known to cause chest pain, migraines, depression, skin rashes, hives, heart irregularities, asthma, seizures, nausea, itching, and headaches in a number of cases and reports.

How You Can Protect Yourself From Media Consumption

Now that you are aware of what goes on behind the scenes in the food industry, how, then, can you protect yourself from being tempted? When it comes to enticing us to give in to our urges and binges, media plays a monumental role in society. More than 80% of Americans watch television every day, averaging approximately over three hours daily. The youth are actually more susceptible, averaging about seven and a half hours every day on some form of media—that's already a third of a whole day. Mass media significantly influences not only how we perceive ourselves and our body image, but also what we want—or *think* we want—to consume. Body ideals and self-value can also be dictated by media, as well as sending a message out there on what should or shouldn't be eaten.

We have already established that the whole "thin" ideal leads to intense body dissatisfaction and eventually to BED. So with all of this media noise around us every waking hour of the day, how can we protect ourselves from unwanted subliminal messages and practice media self-care instead?

1. Be mindful about the media that you choose. Being selective about the kind of things you watch helps you pick out the ones that actually support your values and keeps you from doubting your own body confidence. It helps boost your self-esteem and keeps you from comparing yourself to other people's impossibly high and unrealistic standards, as well as prevents you from bingeing on tempting food you don't actually need. How will you be tempted to indulge in a big, juicy, fat-laden burger if you don't see it on your TV screen every few minutes?

2. Limit the hours you spend on TV and on social media channels. You won't be vulnerable to body concern issues and unhealthy junk food if you don't spend all your time on TV or the internet. Instead, aim for body positivity and reinforce your own ideas.

3. Be more critical about what you see. Are these images digitally altered? Is the gooey goodness of that mozzarella pizza all about camera tricks and proper food photography? Don't let your eyes dictate what your stomach craves for. When bombarded with food advertisements and other commercials, learn how to effectively analyze the carefully crafted message that the media is trying to send out. Remember that these ads are made to convince you to buy a particular product, effectively trying to create an emotional experience for you.

4. Be your own filter. It's important, then, for us to develop our own way to detach ourselves from the ads we see every day. We see what the advertiser wants us to see, but only we alone have the power to control our own media experience. Understand the media message, then assess whether or not you want to believe the message. This is true for both body image and food temptations, so mind your media wisely.

In this chapter, we learned how big multinational food manufacturers create ingenious ways to get consumers addicted to their food. Sugar, salt, and fat, when used in excess, can make any kind of food highly addictive, especially when these foods are readily available and incredibly affordable. Messages we receive on all forms of media also dictate how we react to these impulse food binges, making food as appetizing as possible. To keep from bingeing mindlessly, we have to develop our own filter system wherein we gauge the message that the media is trying to send us, and then properly decide without being driven by our emotions.

Chapter 13: Educate yourself

WHEN I FINALLY started taking my binge eating problem seriously and began my recovery in earnest, I was surprised to find how little I actually knew about binge eating. Over the course of twenty years I had spent endless hours thinking about food and agonising over my binging, and yet I had accumulated very little tangible insight or knowledge.

I hadn't educated myself on the causes of binge eating, I didn't know what treatment options were available or how credible and effective they were, and for a long time I wasn't even aware something called binge eating disorder existed. In short, I was largely ignorant — partly because I chose to be ignorant. Although binge eating was making my life a misery, I didn't want to admit I had a problem, so I didn't bother educating myself.

That was a big mistake. My ignorance cost me lots of time and money because I ended up following idiotic advice and listening to snake oil merchants. Time and again I fell for total BS. I don't want you to be in that same situation, so over the next few pages I'm going to put you through Binge Eating 101. This will give you a grounding in the key fundamentals of binge eating:

- *What is binge eating?*
- *What is binge eating disorder?*
- *What are the signs and symptoms?*
- *What causes binge eating?*
- *What are the treatment options?*

WHAT IS BINGE EATING?

Binge eating (sometimes also called compulsive overeating) involves eating unusually large quantities of food in a short period of time. This is accompanied by one or several of the following signs:

- *Eating very quickly*
- *A sense of loss of control*
- *Feeling as if on autopilot*
- *Feeling dazed*
- *Eating until in physical discomfort or pain*
- *Eating despite being already full or not feeling hungry*
- *Eating in secret*
- *Eating while distracted or carrying out other activities (such as walking)*

- *Feeling guilty, ashamed or depressed afterwards*

In contrast to bulimia, where food binges are followed by purges (typically through vomiting or laxative abuse), binge eaters do not typically purge.

There is no official definition for how large the quantities need to be in order to qualify as a binge or what exactly 'a short period of time' is. I have seen some therapists and coaches talk about 3,000 calories as a typical binge size, but that's anecdotal evidence only and open to debate.

The important point is that we're not talking about having an extra helping of dessert or two chocolate bars instead of one; neither are we talking about regular overeating throughout the day. Binge eating involves amounts of food that are much larger than what most people would consider normal, and the binges take place in a relatively condensed time window (for example one or two hours).

WHAT IS BINGE EATING DISORDER?

When someone binges on a regular basis (typically defined as at least once a week for three months), they may suffer from binge eating disorder (BED).

A BED diagnosis will take into account how often a person binges as well as the impact of the binges on their overall mental health, among other factors. This book can't tell you if you have binge eating disorder or some other form of binge eating problem; only a qualified professional will be able to give you a definitive diagnosis.

That's why I use the more generic term 'binge eating problem' instead of binge eating disorder. In practice, I don't believe the terminology makes much difference to your recovery options, but I want to be clear I am not offering a BED diagnosis here.

Binge eating disorder was officially recognised as an eating disorder in 2013, putting it on a par with anorexia and bulimia, when it was added to the Diagnostic and Statistical Manual of Mental Disorders (DSM-5) of the American Psychiatric Association. This was an important moment, as formal recognition tends to increase awareness in the medical community and means people with binge eating problems are now more likely to be referred to a mental health professional if they seek advice from their family doctor or general practitioner.

Official eating disorder status also means BED is more likely to be of interest to academics and researchers (and they'll find it easier to get funding), which in turn should lead to better treatment options in the future. This can't come soon enough: Although BED was only recently recognised as an eating disorder, it is already considered the most common of all eating disorders, affecting people of all genders, ages, races and ethnic groups.

WHAT ARE THE SIGNS & SYMPTOMS?

You know about the food binges. They are the most obvious and best-known sign of a binge eating problem. However, there's more to binge eating than eating large amounts of food. Two other signs in particular are worth highlighting:

- *Extreme preoccupation with food*
- *Extreme concern about body weight and shape*

Binge eaters tend to be *unusually interested in food*. They spend far more time than most people thinking, reading and talking about food, eating, diets and related subjects. For some binge eaters, this manifests itself in constant worrying about what they've just eaten, whether they ate the right foods or the right amount, what they're going to eat next, if they're going to binge, what they are going to eat if they'll binge, and so on. For others, it can mean actively cultivating interests or seeking out hobbies and past times (and in some cases even occupations) to do with food. This could include cooking for others, watching food shows on TV, spending lots of time researching recipes or looking at food pictures on social media, devising complex diet plans and eating regimens, or even learning about food ethics, sustainability, sourcing and welfare standards.

These are perfectly valid interests and activities for most people, of course, but for binge eaters they can indicate an unhealthy obsession with all things food. Creating more mental space away from food is therefore an important aspect of binge eating recovery. (You'll learn more about this here.)

Another important sign to be aware of is a tendency to be *unusually worried about body shape and weight*. The emphasis here is on *unusually*. Most people are concerned about their size and weight to some extent; lots of people would like to lose weight or change some aspect of their body. Unfortunately, that's the reality of the diet culture that surrounds us. What makes binge eaters different is how much importance they place on body size and weight compared with other people. It's not a small consideration or a minor dissatisfaction. Binge eaters' sense of self-worth, happiness and general achievement in life is completely intertwined with their body image. Losing weight is often the most important goal they feel they need to pursue, and happiness won't be possible if they don't manage to change their body.

This kind of thinking is something binge eating has in common with other eating disorders, and the actual size and weight of the person is irrelevant. Although many binge eaters gain weight as a result of their binges (myself included), not all are medically overweight. Poor body image and obsession with weight loss can happen to people who are a 'normal' weight.

When you plan your own recovery later, it's therefore important you look for strategies that aren't just focused on regulating your eating but address all three key signs of binge eating: The food binges, the obsessive thoughts about food and the poor body image.

This is a tricky question. The short answer is: No one is entirely sure at this stage. As binge eating disorder was only formally recognised in 2013, there hasn't been an awful lot of scientific and academic research to date. Right now there are several different — and at times contradictory — theories to explain what might cause binge eating, including:

- **Genetics**
- *Traumatic childhood events or a history of abuse*
- *Extreme dieting*
- **Depression**
- *Substance abuse*
- *Experience of body shaming or bullying*

For some people all of these factors may play a part in why they develop binge eating problems; for others it might just be one or even none at all. The two main points for you to take away are:

- *There are still lots of unanswered questions about binge eating*
- *It's likely that multiple factors play a role*

So whenever some self-appointed binge eating 'expert' claims to have identified THE ONE THING that is causing you to binge (*Sugar! Carbs! Body hate!*) it's a good idea to be sceptical. They're probably overstating their case.

Having said this, there is broad agreement on one key point: Food restriction (aka dieting) is a factor for the majority of binge eaters. It may not be the *only* factor, but it plays a role in most cases. That is why credible coaches, therapists and self-help programmes will tell you to stop restricting and dieting while you are working on your recovery from binge eating. And it's why you should be wary of anyone who recommends a diet to you — as a binge eater, restriction is highly likely to harm you.

Why Diets Are So Damaging

Let's start by quickly running through the fundamentals of weight loss. Weight loss happens when your body burns more calories than you're taking in. This is known as a caloric deficit, and creating one requires you to restrict your eating in some way. (Theoretically, you can go into caloric deficit by increasing your physical activity while keeping your eating the same, but most people vastly underestimate just how much extra activity would be needed to achieve this. Therefore, in 99.9% of cases, losing weight requires restricting your food intake.)

Being in a caloric deficit isn't much fun, which is why people look for strategies to make the process more manageable. Enter the diet. Diets are, in essence, strategies to help people achieve a caloric deficit. Those strategies can involve restriction in different ways. Some diets focus primarily on restricting the *amount* of food you consume, for example through counting calories or macros. Others restrict the *types* of food you eat, such as low-fat, low-carb, paleo or keto diets. Others still restrict *when* you eat, for example intermittent fasting, 5:2 dieting, 'no food after 7pm' rules or similar. Whatever it is, the ultimate goal remains the same: Restricting intake enough to create a caloric deficit. Because without the deficit, there's no weight loss. How you achieve that deficit doesn't matter. You could lose weight eating nothing but cake, provided the amount you eat puts you in a caloric deficit.

Restriction, as we've seen, is an integral part of weight loss. The problem is, it's also *a huge trigger for binge eating*. Pretty much all binge eating experts agree on this, even if they disagree considerably in other areas. What makes restriction so problematic are several physiological and psychological factors. It begins with a powerful survival instinct. Your body has, over the course of millennia, been programmed to protect you from starving to death. It sees a caloric deficit as dangerous. *Food is scarce! You're starving!* If you're consistently eating less than you need (i.e., you're in a deliberate deficit because you want to lose weight), sooner or later your body will go into panic mode and try to force you to take in more food. You'll experience this as a strong urge to eat.

Initially you might be able to resist this urge through willpower, but the longer your body believes you're in danger of starving, the stronger the urge will become. Similarly, the stricter the diet and the more aggressive the deficit, the quicker your body will try to fight back by giving you strong eating urges. At some point, these will overwhelm you and you'll do what your body wants — eat enough so the deficit is eradicated.

This urge to eat in response to restriction is not unique to binge eaters. It's what happens to most people when they try to lose weight. They go on a diet, they experience urges, they work hard to keep the urges in check, but at some point the urges overwhelm them. They break the diet and come out of deficit, often by eating larger-than-usual amounts of food, and may even end up heavier than they started. For the average person this experience is disappointing, but ultimately they move on with their life. Perhaps they'll try another diet in a few months' time and see if they have more success then. The worst-case scenario is they become a bit of a yo-yo dieter.

For someone with binge eating tendencies, however, it's a catastrophe. That's because binge eaters tend to put much more importance on body size and weight than 'normal' people. They spend more time than average thinking about their weight, and they are much more likely to see their happiness and success in life as linked to the way their body looks. A failed weight loss attempt therefore isn't a minor blip; it's a crushing defeat that feels life-ruining.

This is the psychological fuel that sets the binge eating wheels in motion. Because now a second powerful urge comes into play: The urge to lose weight at all cost. This urge is what makes a binge eater jump right back into dieting after a binge.

So they restrict food to create a deficit, and soon enough alarm bells start going off in their body once more. *We're starving again! We need food — now!* No prizes for guessing what happens next. This is how you end up in what is called a diet-binge cycle, where you are constantly either on a diet or in a binge phase.

The important thing to realise is this only happens because *both physiological and psychological urges* are present. Someone who goes on a diet and ends up overeating or binging but doesn't have a crippling psychological need to lose weight won't experience the urge to keep restricting their food. Someone who hates their body but doesn't ever restrict their food won't experience the physical urge to binge.

It's the combination of the urge to eat (caused by restriction) and the urge to lose weight (through restriction) that creates the toxic feedback loop of binge eating.

Other Factors

What I've just described is the most commonly accepted explanation for how binge eating starts for most people: Poor body image coupled with restrictive dieting.

However, there are other theories and factors that can explain how binge eating patterns develop. For example, some researchers have found a possible genetic component that could make certain people more prone to developing binge eating. Similarly, a predisposition towards certain mental health problems, such as anxiety or depression, may place some people at greater risk of having a binge eating problem.

Other theories focus on the psychological root causes that contribute to binge eating. These can include childhood trauma or abuse; experiences of body shaming and weight stigma; and problematic role models in the family (such parents who were unhappy with their own weight and frequently engaged in diet talk). Wider diet culture and societal pressures to conform to specific standards of beauty can, of course, also play a role.

Some people find it very illuminating to trace their body image and self-esteem issues back to specific events or to contextualise them in this way, and this kind of analysis can end up being a very useful component of their binge eating recovery. For others (myself included) it's interesting but not that useful in practice. As I explained in the introduction, I understood my mum's own body image issues played a role in my binge eating, but that knowledge didn't help me do anything about my binges.

Crucially, those other theories still assume food restriction plays a role in the vast majority of cases. That is to say, someone with a genetic predisposition for binge eating would *not* go on to develop binge eating if they never restricted their food intake – i.e., if they never went on a diet. And someone who suffered weight stigma would not go on to start binging if they didn't also try to restrict their food intake first.

No matter which way you look at it, restriction is the common factor in almost every explanatory model around binge eating. Therefore, any credible attempt at recovery must tackle food restriction as a matter of priority.

Chapter 14: Do You Have A Binge Eating Problem?

Many publications regarding BED go immediately from defining the disorder to instructing the reader of the consequences and cures. However, few publications address the root causes of BED, which is what this book will venture to explain in this chapter. Unless we know why we end up surrounded by empty bags of food, we cannot discover how to avoid the situation.

Identify Your Emotions

Those who suffer from BED generally have complex relationships with food and themselves. Take a moment to consider how you feel about food; do you regard it is it a means of dealing with stress, an obstacle to your goals, or a necessary evil? Whatever the reason may be, determine whether or not it is a healthy one. Furthermore, how does the consumption of food make you feel about yourself? As confusing and fragile as these relationships may be, they are usually the result of more deeply seeded issues that sometimes involve childhood trauma, mood disorders, or harmful familial relationships. Seek help from a medical professional such as a therapist or psychiatrist to deal with these issues at the heart of your disorder and help you towards a healthier mental, emotional, and physical state. In the meantime, begin your own self-analysis by taking stalk of your emotions immediately prior to a binge eating session.

When you feel yourself getting ready to begin a binging episode, try to take a moment to pause. Ask yourself, how am I feeling? This is often the first step towards helping yourself. Many who binge eat report feeling stress, shame, guilt, anger, or a number of other emotions as catalysts for episodes. Once you have identified your emotion, ask yourself why you are feeling that way. As stated earlier, while many of the reasons for binge eating are directly related to previous binge eating episodes, there are often deeper reasons involved. Some studies have found that those afflicted with BED may have been bullied or even sexually assaulted. BED has also been linked to mental disorders (i.e. depression, anxiety, or personality disorders), trouble coping with feelings, and poor impulse control.[2] If you have experienced any of these in the past, dealing with these issues will be a key first step to keeping yourself from binge eating. This is why it is so vital to see professional help at the start of your recovery: there are many complex elements to BED and it is incredibly difficult for an individual to handle the entire scope of the problem alone. Receiving professional help will greatly increase your chances for success and allow a measure of relief from the burden of BED.

Another important aspect to be aware of is the type of binges you partake in. Some people binge purely at night in order to either hide their eating habits or to make up for the severe dieting they have been doing in the daytime, thus overcompensating for the lack of nutrition their bodies are incurring. Others deal with another type of secret binging, in which they rearrange their schedules in order to be alone during times they wish to binge. In contrast to this type of planned binging, impulsive binging is also very common, in which the consumer immediately begins binging due to a particular mood or event that may have just occurred.

It is important to realize that an individual's particular type of binging and reason for binging are related to one another. Find the reason why you partake in a certain method of binging and identify the emotion related to it. Then you will be able to take steps towards dealing with those emotions and confronting their root causes. Again, this kind of self-analysis can be very difficult and often bring up pent up feelings that may have fermenting for several years. As the clinical psychologist Dr. Mary Froning, Psy.D., said, "Binge eating is literally stuffing feelings down" (Editors, *Are You a Binge Eater*).[3] Identify those feelings that are causing your behavior and you'll be one step closer eradicating it.

Understand Your Thoughts

Once you have dealt with the problem of identifying your emotions in regards to binge eating, it is time to interpret your feelings directly before beginning a binge. It's possible that some people begin binging simply because they think they are hungry, when in fact they are thirsty. Not only does this lead to extreme overeating, but also to dehydration, which further hurts the body and mind. Dr. Harris Lieberman, Ph.D., found that even a small amount of dehydration that lasts between 4-8 hours significantly affects the mind and body. Specifically, those who are dehydrated are apt to feel more tired and have a worsened mood.[4] If this is the case for you, then the lack of water may be contributing to your disorder.

However, a problem that may be more common is mistaking hunger for anger, boredom, or depression. It is important to recognize these emotions early on, before reaching for the refrigerator or pantry. If you realize, either before or during a binge, the real reason for the food rampage, stop and pause. Realize that your body does not need the food and that the craving is related to satisfying a feeling rather than hunger. Consider writing down what you are feeling or speaking with a friend, relative, or a medical professional to discuss these feelings.

In time, you may begin to discover a pattern. It may be that every time you go to begin a binge eating session, you feel guilty or ashamed. Recognizing a trigger feeling and when it occurs may assist with stopping binge eating episodes before they begin. Hopefully, you will also be able to avoid the circumstances that make you feel those emotions in the future.

While these patterns are good ones to observe, they may not apply to you. Many people plan out their binges, making sure to be at home in solitude so they can eat without distractions. For these types of situations, it is equally important to identify and understand your emotions, but not place extreme emphasis on impulse control. Determine for yourself what it is about your life or self that makes you act out in this way. Realizing that perhaps you have a negative outlook on life or yourself may help you to begin changing your outlook and thus cut off binging sessions before they happen. Take into careful consideration how you perceive other binge eaters and how your peers and family view you or food. This may speak volumes as to your relationship with yourself. If you perceive other binge eaters or perhaps obese individuals negatively, try to change your attitude by regarding them with compassion. This may in turn help you to view yourself and food in a more positive light. However, if you suspect family members or friends, due to shame and/or criticism, are the cause of your negative feelings, it would be wise to have a frank discussion with and perhaps distance yourself from those individuals. Have a talk with your therapist about the best way to approach these conversations.

Now comes the question of keeping yourself from binging once you have recognized that you want to begin overeating. This can be very difficult because, usually, there is always food in the house and even getting in your car allows access to grocery stores, fast food chains, and restaurants. So it is important to be able to take your mind off of food entirely. How is this possible? Psychologist Dr. Dori Winchell, Ph.D., tells us "Once you are engaged in a task you enjoy and must pay attention to, you're less likely to be fixated on food" (Editors, *Are You a Binge Eater*).[5] So when you do not feel like eating, find a task that you truly enjoy, preferably something that is not high-maintenance or requires a lot of travel, as something on hand will be easier to gain access to when feelings of binging come on. Try something like a game of Sudoku, running, or gardening. As long as it keeps your mind off of food and your body out of the kitchen, it should help with the food cravings. One thing to be sure not to substitute food for, however, is another addiction. Be wary of trading food binges for a cigarette, a drink, shopping at the mall, or even extreme exercise. These activities may keep you from overeating but will only help to fuel addictive traits. Remember, helping yourself is not about stopping the binge eating, but changing thought patterns and dealing with emotions in a healthy manner.

Don't Do It Alone

In many cases, binge eaters suffer alone, hiding their disorder even from close friends and family. Carrying a weight as heavy as a disorder causes enormous stress for the individual, which can further fuel binge eating. If you are someone who hides their disorder from the world, it is time to have an honest discussion with your family and friends.

This is not to say that everyone needs to know you about your situation, nor is the admission meant to place any sort of blame upon you. Rather, having a open talk with people you trust aims to alleviate much of the stress caused by keeping such a huge secret. If one of the keys to continuing BED over long periods of time is keeping the behavior to yourself, than an essential element to recovery is admitting your condition to others and trusting them to help you. By letting others into this delicate part of your life, you open yourself up to support. This support should be taken advantage of as often as needed and comes in the form of various resources. Begin by telling a select number of friends and family about your disorder and that you are beginning on your path to a healthier you. Ask for their support and impress your need for their care and consideration. After this, seek out additional helpful resources; contact a medical professional who can aid you with therapy sessions or monitor your health as you improve. If reaching out to others for help is particularly difficult for you, consider consulting a medical professional first in order to address the root causes regarding your lack of comfort when asking for help. Take whatever route is easiest for you, as long as it moves you forward instead of keeping you stagnant. Also consider researching groups in your area or online forums with members who have experienced similar problems. If all of this sounds intimidating, don't worry. Many resources will be listed later in this book to help you create your safety net.

Perhaps all of this is sounding a bit extreme. If this is the case, allow this to stand as a motivating reminder: BED can and will severely reduce your quality of life if left unchecked, and may very well reduce your life span. Binge eating often results in joint pain, high cholesterol, obesity, depression, severe anxiety, heart disease, and increased risk for strokes. This is not even taking into account the toll it takes on relationships, whether that be because you are keeping a huge part of your life a secret from loved ones, because BED has led to weight problems and the idea of playing with your child is exhausting, or even because you cannot accept an invitation to a meal for fear of being unable to prevent a binge eating episode.

In spite of these harsh facts, it is nourishing to know that the rewards of ceasing binge eating habits can be remarkable. Imagine what it would be like to make plans to go traveling across the country with friends without fear of food or to run around a playground with your child. Imagine how it would feel to just wake up in the morning and not already be exhausted by the thought of the coming day. This is why you must strive to rid yourself of BED; so that life will be open to you with all of it's possibilities, and you will be free to take them.

Chapter 15: How to Create a Healthy Lifestyle That Supports Your Recovery

In this chapter, we will learn about the different hobbies that you can get into during recovery. We will also discuss the right mindset and attitude you should have toward exercise, and why it's important to pick the right activity that's best for you.

Various Hobbies That Can Improve Your Ability to Cope

Hobbies are extremely beneficial to your emotional health and overall well-being. With people who suffer from Binge Eating Disorder, oftentimes, it might feel like there is a total loss of self. Patients might feel empty inside, usually unable to see their self-worth. Finding new hobbies and coping skills can be quite a challenge, but once you find one that best suits your lifestyle and your personality, the result is immensely satisfying.

There are many types of hobbies that you can try on your road to recovery. Hiking is a good choice if you are more into the outdoors, as it is always a good idea to immerse yourself in nature every chance you get. If you are looking for an activity that's more emotionally focused and meditative, you can go for a yoga practice and its many variations. Even the simple act of walking can already be relaxing and restorative, especially if you make this a hobby and have a few friends tag along with you.

Group hobbies help you slowly get back out there on a social scale. Usually, if you engage in activities with like-minded individuals or those who are also focused on recovery, you will be able to successfully shift your focus from your bingeing thoughts to more positive ones about your body. You can even work together and support one another—all while having fun in the process.

It is very important during this stage to never stop rediscovering who you are. Take a few moments to reflect on the activities you enjoyed prior to your BED, and try to asses if everything is still the same, or if things have changed. Are there any particular activities that you would like to try now along with your peers? Are there any new skills you learned during therapy that you would like to try out? Did you engage in an art therapy session once and find that it's actually something that you really like doing? Does knitting relax you, or does cooking spark something inside you that brings joy to your day? It's always scary to try new things, but most worthwhile things often are—you never know what activity out there will ignite a passion in you that you never knew existed.

And while you're at it, why not schedule a weekly breakfast or meet up with your peers to check on how everyone is doing? This way, you can be held accountable during your recovery, and at the same time help support others who might be getting off-track. The important thing is to keep trying and to keep discovering. Do not be afraid to open up to your family and friends, and even enlist them to join you on your new hobby. Who knows? You just might start a new tradition among your loved ones beginning today.

Learn the best hobby that suits you personally. There is no one-size-fits-all hobby, but here are just some things you need to keep in mind to help boost your metabolism rate and speed up your recovery:

1. *Do not judge yourself.* Be open to new things, and let go of your old ways of thinking. People who suffer from BED often believe that exercise during BED

recovery means weight loss. Due to this unhealthy way of thinking, they often push themselves to the limit and try to exert themselves excessively. Instead, you need to make peace with what your body can and cannot do. Forget all of the "shoulds" and "need to's". Open yourself up to the idea that you can build a good relationship with exercise without worrying too much about calories and statistics. Listen to your body, and rest when you are tired. Exercise can be fun in itself, so gently tell your mind to let go of its anxieties and just enjoy.

2. You cannot achieve recovery all alone. It's imperative that you let others in—whether it's a loved one or someone who is going through the same things you are. Recovery is extremely challenging, and having someone to lean on as your safety net when things get too difficult is mandatory. During this serious struggle, you can bring back exercise into your life with the support of your loved ones and your team of professionals, so that you can experience working out in a peaceful way that's filled with joy and balance.

3. It's okay to be honest. If you feel like exercise is causing you even more anxiety than helping you, talk to your treatment specialists about it. Be honest with your intentions, and more importantly, be honest with yourself. Do not let your weight define you; nor should you try to be "perfect" all the time. Remember that your physical exercise should have a positive effect on your emotional and mental health as well, so if it throws your body out of whack or doesn't promote body balance, then perhaps that particular exercise is not for you.

Types of Physical Exercises and Their Benefits

More than looking for a hobby that you will actually enjoy, finding the right workout to help boost your metabolism and facilitate your recovery is also crucial.

1. Cardio training (aerobic and anaerobic)

As one of the most popular types of exercises, cardio has a ton of varieties that you can try out to see what works best for you. You can go running, walking, cycling, swimming, dancing—the possibilities are endless. The basic idea is to get your heart rate up and elevate it to a level above your normal resting rate.

Aerobic or steady state cardio means that you are aiming for a steady pace and intensity during your workout. Your breathing and heart rate speed up to increase endurance and to help you walk up those flights of stairs without breaking a sweat. This type of exercise helps condition your lungs and your heart, as well as help your muscles work more efficiently as enough blood is pumped into them. Aside from this, your blood vessel walls also learn to relax, and as you burn fat, you also lower your blood sugar levels and your blood pressure. You raise both the good cholesterol (or HDL cholesterol) and your mood. In the long run, you help reduce your risk of stroke, heart disease, breast cancer, colon cancer, depression, and type 2 diabetes.

Low and moderate intensity aerobic exercise means that your heart rate remains below half of your Maximum Heart Rate (MHR). For moderate intensity workouts, your heart rate stays between 50% to approximately 70% of your MHR. This includes activities like biking, running, swimming, fitness classes, and hiking—you should still be able to talk with someone and carry out a conversation. For high intensity (anaerobic) workouts, you push your heart rate to a higher intensity, keeping it to above 70% of your MHR. This includes what is known as HIIT (high-intensity interval training), which means that your exercises are efficiently separated into "intervals" or repetitions within rounds. With this kind of workout, you should always remember to keep your work-to-rest ratio. For beginners, aim for a 1:2 ratio of one part high-intensity and then two parts low-intensity interval. This lets your body recover properly during "breaks" before you start up the high-intensity workout again.

As an average, you can try to make 150 minutes of moderate intensity activity your weekly goal. One of the simplest things you can do while you are starting out is to simply march in place. Begin your starting position by standing tall with your arms at your sides and your feet together. Then, slowly bend your elbows and swing your arms, just as you lift up your knees at the same time. Tighten your abs, look ahead, and breathe at a comfortable pace. You can even march about four steps forward and then backward, or alternate between marching with your feet together and then with your feet wide apart—whichever works best for you.

2. Strength training

Regular strength training builds back any muscle mass lost as we age. Do not mistake strength training as suited only for weight lifters and athletes—this type of exercise also helps you carry out simple day-to-day tasks such as gardening, carrying your groceries, and even getting up from the floor.

It makes you stronger, lowers blood sugar, stimulates your bone growth, enhances your posture, improves your balance, and reduces pain in your joints and in your lower back. It also reduces stress overall, so don't be afraid to ask your therapist which activity works best for you. You can do push-ups, lunges, or squats. Simply stand with your arms at your sides and your feet about shoulder width apart. Then, bend your knees and your hips, lower your buttocks to approximately eight inches or so, and balance your body by swinging your arms forward. Remember to keep your back straight, shift your weight over to your heels, and repeat as necessary.

3. Flexibility training

What does flexibility mean to you? Is it being able to twist your torso around, or is it the ability to touch your toes? More than just expanding your range of motion, flexibility is all about your overall musculoskeletal health. There are plenty of exercises that help boost your mobility and flexibility to help prevent injury later on, so if you are not naturally born with it, all hope isn't lost. Just remember to keep an open mind whenever you are doing your flexibility training, as even the simple act of stretching can already bring you closer to your fitness goals even though the exertion seems minimal at the beginning.

With static stretching, you develop your muscular tension by holding a position for about half a minute. The position should be challenging enough but without contracting your muscles. When you repeatedly move through a range of motion, you are dynamically stretching. Passive stretching, on the other hand, means that you are relaxing into a stretch with the help of an external force. This external assistance can be a person or a tool that helps intensify the stretch. With active stretching, you relax the muscle you are stretching, and then depend on an opposing muscle during motion.

Proper stretching can reduce the risk of injury, falling, strains, joint pain, muscle damage, muscle cramps, and other muscle pains that come with age. It can help you function properly in daily life, such as when bending down or even just to tie your shoelaces. It's a good goal to stretch every day, first warming up your muscles with dynamic stretches and then holding challenging positions for about a minute with static stretches. Static stretches can be done with your hamstrings, calves, quadriceps, hip flexors, quadriceps, shoulders, and neck. Just remember not to stretch to a point where you start to feel pain. This tightens your muscles even further, which is not the goal of stretching.

Try a single knee rotation when you're starting out. First, lie on your back and extend your legs on the floor. Second, relax both your shoulders against the floor as well. Then, bend your left knee slowly, positioning your left foot over on your right thigh (aim for the spot just above the knee). Remember to keep your abdominal muscles tight. When you can, go ahead and use your right hand to gently pull your left knee to your right side. Hold for half a minute.

Another good suggestion for flexibility and mobility is yoga. You can choose from Ashtanga, Hatha, Iyengar, Vinyasa flow, hot yoga, or yin. These yoga practices help integrate your body and your breath; plus, they help you practice mindfulness as you become aware of your body with each flow. With a regular yoga practice, you can loosen and mobilize your joints, stretch your ligaments, enhance your muscle strength, keep you nice and limber, and boost your flexibility as well.

4. Balance training

The ability to stay balanced keeps you from falling and reduces the risk of injury. When we get older, our inner ear, our leg muscles, and our vision all slowly break down, making us more susceptible to falling down. Training your balance only ensures that you maintain your steadiness as you grow with age. In fact, a lot of senior centers offer classes that enhance balance like yoga or tai chi—even if you don't have any issues with your own balance, it's still a good idea to start early and train your steadiness.

Different kinds of balance training exercises include standing on one foot, walking on surfaces that are uneven, and strengthening your leg muscles with leg lifts and squats. Beginners can first try a simple standing knee lift, wherein you stand with your feet together. Keep your hands on your hips, then slowly lift your knee. Lift it toward the ceiling as high as you can, as comfortably as you can. Aim to keep your thigh parallel to the floor, but remember not to overexert yourself. It can take some time to get used to this position, so do not try to push yourself too hard, especially if you are just starting out. Hold the position as long as you can, then lower back down to your starting position. Repeat as necessary with your other leg. Remember to tighten your abs and keep your shoulders down and back. Lift your chest, and tighten your buttocks to keep steady. To help you with your stability, you can opt to hold on to a chair or a countertop with one hand until you can balance without any external support.

In this chapter, we learned that learning different hobbies can help you take back your life while recovering from BED. There are a variety of exercises to choose from to speed up your metabolism and boost your recovery. Cardio reduces your blood pressure, improves your cardio-respiratory health, enhances your pulmonary wellbeing, and improves circulation. Weight training enhances your strength, endurance, and muscle mass, as well as increases your bone density and strengthens your joints. Flexibility and balance training improve your range of motion, boosts your spinal musculoskeletal wellbeing, helps you release physical and mental tension, and lowers the risk of injury and falls.

Chapter 16: Movement Instead of Exercise

Working out at the gym is a familiar routine for many people. Exercise is a great way to keep in shape and healthy. Yoga, weightlifting, cycling, swimming and many other activities are ideal for staying fit. Some people may experience exercise in a very positive way, whether its competitive or challenging (team sports, martial arts) or self-improving through individual training and coaching. Other people may view exercise as a necessary evil or chore, especially if they experience pain or discomfort from chronic conditions, injuries, or do not find exercise enjoyable at all. There is another way to look at exercise: Movement. Movement shifts all the stress of what exercise means to a more inclusive approach of overall betterment. When most people think of exercise, they may only perceive it in a limited way, like spending time in the gym doing repetitive cardiovascular movements and weights. These perceptions may include team sports or specific types of routines, while the definition of movement widens to capture walking, dancing, stretching and basically any form of motion that improves mobility and fitness. It is also more inclusive of people with varying abilities and who may not otherwise be able to participate in regular fitness programs. As with intuitive eating gives mindfulness to the way we eat, the movement does the same for the way we stay in shape.

Mindful movement is a great way to extend the benefits of intuitive eating to overall health. When we exercise, we focus on our body and in many cases, we target certain parts of our bodies for results: losing weight in our abdominal area with core stretches, weight training for muscles, running and cycling for burning calories. These are all positive activities, though we often do them without paying attention to how they impact our bodies. A long run can impact your knees or a strenuous routine and excessive movement can pull muscles if overdone. Mindful movement engages the mind and thoughts into the body, to actively connect your breathing, mental focus, and physical movement together.

There are significant benefits, in conjunction with intuitive or mindful eating. The results are similar for different ages of people, with the outcome usually the same: lower levels of stress, better cardiovascular health, and less anxiety. Taking deep, measured breaths during yoga and similar movement exercise (including Pilates), can improve your circulation and lower your stress within a short period of time. When we feel stress, we breathe shallow or hold our breath. This can contribute to anxiety. Breathing deeply while we meditate or stretch and pose, takes away that tension we build on in our bodies. When you relax, food cravings resulting from stress or emotion will fall away, leaving you only wanting to eat if you are truly hungry, therefore engaging intuitive eating as well.

Focus improves when you meditate and practice mindful movement. This will improve your performance in work, life, and mental awareness, helping you become successful at decision making and more balanced. Getting started is as easy as finding a forest or park outdoors, where you can walk, stretch or cycle. In some cities, groups of people enjoy practicing yoga or tai chi outdoors. Joining a group is a great way to meeting people with similar goals, though these exercises are just as enjoyable solo and a good way to empty your thoughts and clear your mind. Joining a local yoga or Pilates class is another way to begin mindful exercise. Try a beginner yoga class, if you are new to this practice. If you experience chronic pain or have a condition that requires modified techniques, try a restorative yoga class or discuss with an experienced yoga instructor in advance. Often, a few modifications, if any, are all that's needed to enjoy yoga. Once you begin to practice regularly, you'll notice more flexibility, less anxiety and a sense of peace. Some classes offer meditation during or following a session of yoga. There are also different levels and types of yoga that may be helpful to research beforehand, such as "hatha," or Vinyasa yoga.

Yoga is very beneficial in combination with mindful eating and living. There are many poses, movements, and modifications that can fit your abilities and body. One feature of yoga class is the option to move on your own time, not exactly in sync with the instructor or guide, but rather, in connection with how you feel. The downward dog pose is one of the most popular and common during yoga class. In this pose, your body positioned in a downward "V" shape, with both palms on the floor, shoulder width apart, and your feet on the ground, also the same distance apart. In this shape, you can stretch closer or further apart, lift one leg or arm to stretch, and even practice breathing. Your posture will improve as a result of practicing the downward dog and other poses, such as cat or cow, cobra, and other poses provide many other benefits for your body. There are specific movements and breathing techniques to aid in digestion and relieving pain from indigestion.

Pilates is a set of exercises that focus on core strength, flexibility, and balance. These were developed by Joseph Pilates and has become very popular in fitness studios. Pilates, like yoga, can be modified to accommodate a range of abilities, as the movements are graceful and easy to learn. The practice is beneficial in relieving stress, improving circulation and is a bit more intense than yoga. Pilates is great for strengthening your core, abdominals and pelvic region, which is gentle, yet effective in post-partum and in feeling well overall.

Both Yoga and Pilates have many variations, and it's worth trying several different styles to find the best fit for you. Pilates can be more demanding on the body, so if you are new to these types of movements, begin slowly. Try yoga first and discuss any physical restrictions or conditions that may impact your motion.

There are always modifications to help you maximize the most out of your workout.

The Motivation for Starting Intuitive Eating
Most, if not all, people who diet will try more than one diet in their lifetime. Think of how many types of eating habits or ways of dieting you have tried, even if briefly. With every way of eating, there are self-described experts, authors, recipes, and guides. Almost every grocery checkout lane showcases magazines with new ways to lose ten pounds in a week or other ways to lose weight fast. For each diet, you may have tried more than one method, slipped a few times, only to restart or change again. There are options to combine diets, from intermittent fasting and low carb eating, to paleo vegetarian or macrobiotic. There are many possibilities and options, and all of them require a lot of effort and time. Intuitive eating puts the focus on your body, as an individual and your needs, above all else. When you focus on what you need, the signals your body sends, there is less effort on following a set of rules and more on what is nutritious and good for you.

There are many reasons to abandon dieting for mindful eating, including:

1.*Putting an end to chronic dieting*. Even the most successful diets are destined to fail because there is no one-size-fits-all for every individual. Shifting from one diet to another only reaffirms this. Leaving diets behind will also eliminate all the stress associated with it

2.*Individualizing your way of eating.* Diets assume, for the most part, that people can "fit" into one method for results. This is inaccurate, considering the variety of body types, metabolism levels, health conditions, and the environment. Mindful eating focuses on you getting to know your body and what it needs.

3.*Breaking the cycle of programming.* From early on, we are told what to eat, and how much. A palm size of carbohydrates, a fist full of protein and heaps of vegetables. Food groups and charts have been promoted over decades at schools and doctor's offices. Eating well cannot be defined by a chart, as with diets, everyone is an individual with their own needs.

4.*Consistency.* Foods that are listed as unhealthy years ago (think fats) are now considered healthy, whereas sugar and salt are either overused or completely avoided altogether. Coffee, wine and coconut oil are either beneficial or unhealthy for you, depending what source you read. Mindful eating doesn't categorize or rate foods, keeping the choice completely up to your discretion.

5. *Overall better connection to your mind and body.* Reduced stress, better focus, and decision making when it comes to eating means less overindulging and more enjoyment of food and the way we eat.

6. *Increased confidence.* Intuitive eating practices have shown a positive impact on how we view and treat our bodies. The more we become connected to our inner needs and body, the more respect we have for ourselves. This results in a better feeling about our image and setting realistic expectations.

7. *Taking away the compulsion to eat "bad" foods and viewing them as occasional treats.* When you eat according to your individual needs and no foods are forbidden, as they are all considered equally. The result is this: no guilt for eating certain foods means we don't feel a compulsion to binge on them.

We live in a society where we are constantly aware of our image and of those around us. We are also inundated with a lot of expectations and place a lot of pressure on ourselves to fit a level of expectation, which is often unrealistic. This causes perfectionism, which is unattainable and results in lower self-esteem and confidence. By changing the dynamic from meeting these unreasonable expectations and working from within and following our individual needs, a healthier pattern emerges with lasting positive effects.

Beginning Your Journey to Mindful Eating

There are many sources to read for support and ideas on how to start your new way of eating. These can be helpful for people who prefer direction on where to begin. Where do I start? Once I recognize my hunger and want to eat, how do I enjoy my meal and continue from there? A strong foundation for successful intuitive eating will begin by employing the following basics:

1. *Take time to enjoy your meal.* Don't rush your lunch. If you are in a hurry, eat a healthy snack if you are hungry and wait until you have at least half an hour to relax. Reduce other tasks during this break to maximize your time. Eat slowly, chew every mouthful carefully, intentionally, savoring the flavor and texture of the food. If you normally eat out for lunch, choose a quiet section of the restaurant or café. If you are in a cafeteria at work, find an area with the least amount of noise and distraction, and if it's too loud or busy,

choose a quiet place outside in a park where you can relax. This will help you achieve satisfaction and maximize your experience with food.

2. *Avoid distractions and eliminate excessive food.* When you eat with others, try to plan your meal ahead so that there is little room for decision making when you order. Bring your own food or find out what's on the menu before your meal. This will take the pressure of making impulsive choices in the moment, such as choosing too much food that can't be enjoyed or not enough. If you're meeting at a restaurant, call ahead or check out the menu online to find out what's available. Focus on socializing, enjoying food and leave the stress behind!

If you eat alone, savor the meal in silence or with gentle sounds of music or nature. Avoid your phone, television and other distractions. Let your food take center stage so that it can be consumed and relished fully.

3. *Focus on your hunger level.* As you eat, pay attention to how you feel. Eating slowly allows for better digestion. It can take up to twenty minutes to realize you are full, so taking your time is best. Once you are full, stop eating and relax. Don't rush away;

drink some water, tea or simply stop, in order to allow your body to adjust. Realizing you are full is the key to staying in tune with your body's signals. Hours later, you will feel hungry again, though it may only require a light meal, depending on how long you wait and how often you eat. A pattern will form and listening to your body's signals will get easier with time.

4. *Pay attention to your emotions.* When you eat, how do you feel? If you are anxious or upset, you may eat a lot more and faster than expected. This will lead to indigestion and feeling unwell hours later. You may find that concentration and being active become more challenging after you overeat. It will also have a significant effect on your mood, and this is how synching our body's signals with our needs are very important in curbing unexpected changes in our moods, energy levels, and performance. When you eat, is it because you're hungry? Or is it a response to something else? Are you eating due to an emotional response? Or due to boredom? Being aware of these reasons can help turn our attention to dealing with these aspects in our life differently, and instead, reserving eating for when we are truly hungry.

When you eat, do you suddenly feel elated or more anxious? If we make poor food choices, that are not nutritious; we may feel worse after we eat, thinking of the effects on our health. Food is often used as comfort or a vice to ignore or escape from problems in our life, instead of facing them head-on. It's also good to realize that eating something that may not be healthy, on occasion, is not going to undo or stop our success. Intuitive eating can be successful in spite of those experiences and as we become more used to listening to our bodies, it will become less frequent over time. Eating should be enjoyable and nourishing, not stressful or addictive. Mindful eating aims to bring non-hunger reasons for eating into focus so that we can consciously realize when it is appropriate to eat, and when it is not.

5. *Recognize your cravings.* We all experience cravings, even when we're not hungry. Be mindful of them and recognize that they are outside of your signals. If you find cravings to be tempting, take a moment to find a peaceful space and relax. Meditation, even if for a few minutes, can be helpful in relief, as the cravings will pass. Focus on something that will take your mind off of the food or the taste you crave. Enjoy a peaceful

moment in the park, lying or sitting down on a mat or comfortable chair. Facing this sensation and letting it pass through mindfulness is a key part of intuitive eating.

6. *Focus on one meal at a time.* We have busy lives and this involves planning ahead for multiple meals over several days or weeks. This is absolutely necessary to stay within a budget but shouldn't become overwhelming. Keep meals simple and easy to prepare. Visit local markets and eat fresh as much as possible. Start with one meal and focus on the impact of the food you choose. Eliminate food choices that leave you unsatisfied or unwell and refine your options to increase satisfaction more each time. This will help individualize your eating habits for you.

Overall, intuitive eating aims to end dieting and emotional eating, for a better and more mindful, research-based approach to eating and feeling well. This will achieve better health emotionally, psychologically and physically. In tandem with mindful meditation and movement, intuitive eating becomes a new way of living and enjoying your food and life.

Chapter 17: Tips On How To Prevent A Relapse

After discussing the methods you can use to treat emotional eating and binge eating in the previous chapter, it important to discuss tips that will help prevent a relapse back into your old eating habits. Learning how to prevent a relapse into your old unhealthy eating habits makes it easy for you to follow through with treatment. In this chapter, we will discuss several tips that will help you successfully transit from unhealthy eating habits to healthy ones.

Tips to prevent a relapse

The truth of the matter is recovering from binge eating and emotional eating will not be a walk in the park. It will take effort, time, and persistence to ensure that you get over binge eating and emotional eating disorder and get back control over food. Below are tips that will help prevent a relapse as well as give you the motivation to keep moving forward despite the challenges you face.

1. Have a plan

While still on treatment, it is essential to have a plan that will keep you from reverting to your old unhealthy eating habits. The plan can include a food journal and a meal plan. Having a plan is important for the following reasons:

It helps you track your progress: Having a plan while on treatment for an eating disorder like binge eating helps you track your progress. For instance, having a food journal will help you understand the number of calories you eat daily. It will also make it possible to portion your meals and include healthy snacks. Having a method that makes it easy to track your progress helps you know when you experience a relapse.

It enables you to achieve your objectives: One of the most significant objectives of a plan is enabling you to achieve your objectives. Every individual with an eating disorder has a set of objectives they want to achieve. It does, however, become quite difficult to stick to the objectives they set. However, having a plan is a constant reminder that there is a reason to keep working and sticking to the treatment.

It motivates you to keep going: An excellent plan will have incentives that will make it possible for you to keep working to achieve your objectives. It should motivate you and keep you from losing track even when faced with challenges. Having a plan will motivate you to make the right decisions even when you feel like making all the wrong choices.

How to create a plan

When creating a plan, it is essential to ask yourself the following questions.

- How will your diet plan look like? The answer to this question depends on the schedule your treatment plan has for you. You should also consider the number of meals you desire to eat in a day. Having an eating schedule will make it easy for you to divide calories accordingly and eliminate the possibility of overindulging.

- What type of support do you require? Your support system is also necessary to include in your plan. Having support while trying to succeed in getting back your self-control over food helps you stick to your nutrition and treatment plans without falling off the wagon

• Do you require exercise? This another aspect to consider. However, before you include it as part of your routine, it is important for you to consult your doctor. Becoming physically active makes it easy to lose that weight as well as give your body the energy it requires to keep going.

2. Do not skip your meals

Plenty of relapses among individuals suffering from binge eating and emotional eating disorders happen because of skipping a meal. To avoid relapsing, it is essential to never let yourself get extremely hungry. Extreme hunger will make you overeat during one seating and this may essentially lead to you reverting to your previous unhealthy habits. For people suffering from binge eating and emotional eating disorders, skipping meals will not help you manage this condition.

Skipping meals also has serious effects on people with eating disorders. It affects you physically and mentally as well. The physical effects of skipping meals include increased glucose and sugar levels, abdominal weight gain, and overeating. Psychologically, skipping meals will cause a drastic change in your mood.

Have a reminder: Having constantly been told by society that eating regularly is bad and not eating is good, it is quite easy to also have the same line of thought. However, you are actually much better off eating all your meals rather than skipping them. Having a reminder is one of the ways to ensure you never skip a meal. Eating all your meals is important as it helps you stick to your treatment plans without having a reason to binge eat.

Always plan ahead: We all have those days when our lives are constantly stressful and during those moments, it becomes quite easy to turn to food to uplift your spirit. This can eventually lead to a relapse. Planning your meals is one way of avoiding a relapse. Once you plan your snacks and prep your meals beforehand, it takes away any excuses you give yourself to eat food that may cause you to relapse.

Talk to your doctor: If you cannot stop yourself from skipping meals talk to your doctor or a therapist. They will help you come up with effective ways to ensure you eat healthier and regularly.

Eating on a regular basis will help control your hunger, avoid situations that can lead to binging sessions, and it stops you from feeling hungry. Remember, skipping meals can trigger emotional or binge eating symptoms and this can derail your recovery process.

3. Occasionally treat yourself

Treating yourself occasionally is one to ensure that you stick to your objectives without diverting attention to unhealthy foods. Individuals suffering from binge eating disorder or emotional eating disorder have to divide the food they consume into two categories. The "good" category or the "risky" category. Dividing food in such a manner makes it easy for you to avoid including the risky foods as part of your daily meals.

However, such a division can cause you to relapse to binging and overeating. One of the ways to avoid this from happening is by occasionally treating yourself. Why is it important to treat yourself?

- It helps you remain motivated

According to several research studies, occasionally treating yourself can assist you in staying motivated. Creating specific goals for yourself during your treatment journey and then ensuring that you treat yourself after achieving it, helps you stay motivated to achieve a holistic and healthy approach to dealing with your triggers and emotions rather than turn to food for comfort. In order for you to attain optimal results, ensure that you break down your long-term goals into shorter and more achievable goals. This will make it possible for you to reward yourself when you accomplish the shorter goals.

- It prevents a decrease in your metabolic rate

Another benefit of occasionally rewarding yourself is that it helps in preventing a decrease in your metabolic rate. One of the action treatment plans for people suffering from binge eating disorder or emotional eating disorder is the creation of a meal plan. A majority of foods on meal plans are healthy foods. However, completely eradicating some food types can cause your body to experience a decrease in its metabolic rate. The primary reason for this is because your metabolism (the part of your body responsible for digesting food and helps in its storage and excretion) recognizes the food you consume.

This causes your body to decrease the work your metabolism performs and this may result in you gaining even more weight. Therefore, occasionally treating yourself will not only make it easy for you to lose weight; it also prevents occasional cravings.

- It keeps you from binge eating

Finally, treating yourself from time to time prevents you from falling into a binge episode. Categorizing specific foods as bad is one of the primary reasons why plenty of people relapse when undergoing treatment for an eating disorder. Research has found that people who crave for specific foods and end up preventing themselves from eating them, will end up experiencing emotional eating or binging episodes.

This is because people who crave for specific foods will opt for healthier options and since this will not satisfy their cravings, they end up eating, even more, to attempt to satisfy their craving. However, this would not be the case if they had simply eaten the food their bodies craved for. Therefore, occasionally treating yourself is an effective method of ensuring you stick to your treatment and avoid binging episodes.

Remember, your objective should be to incorporate a wide range of food varieties and eat them in moderation.

4. Stay positive

It is important to remember that there are plenty of challenges when undergoing treatment for binge eating disorder and emotional eating. One of the most common challenges is failing to follow through with the treatment and having to start all over again. Having treated binge eating before, I know how it feels to relapse back to binge eating and have to start treatment all over again. Despite it being tough, staying positive about your success, body shape, and yourself helps you get through the difficult times. What makes positivity a powerful weapon when undergoing treatment for eating disorders?

First, it is important to understand that positivity plays a significant role in your treatment process. Negative thoughts lead to self-defeating actions like overeating, turning to food for comfort, and going off your treatment and nutrition plan. Positive thoughts are empowering and they help you through the entire process of recovery. Berating yourself any time you fail to do something right, focusing on what you did not do, or dreading your meals can lead to you relapsing and going back to unhealthy eating habits.

Secondly, positivity helps you stick to your goals despite the challenges you face. It makes it easy for you to have an attitude that forces you to achieve success despite the challenges you face along the way. Your society, family, or environment cannot influence your attitude. Therefore, strive to have an attitude that will help you stick to your treatment and nutrition despite the challenges you face.

5.Ensure you have a support system

It is hard to ignore the fact that trying to recover from an eating disorder has its difficulties and successes. During each stage of your treatment having people you can depend on during the difficult and challenging times, makes the treatment easier to cope with. You require people who will understand the struggles you go through. You require people who will listen to your fears and offer you an honest opinion on what you should do during the difficult times.

Research studies have shown that people with support systems have better-coping skills, high levels of well-being, and healthier lives. Research also shows that having a support system helps in reducing depression and anxiety. Anxiety and depression are some of the emotions that can lead individuals recovering from binge eating disorder or emotional eating disorder into a relapse. To prevent this from happening, it is essential to have a support system.

Types of support systems

The primary objective of any support system is to reduce the amount of stress you may experience when undergoing the treatment process. Support systems are classified into four categories. These four categories are:

Esteem support: This is a type of support that is expressed in the form of encouragement or confidence. People in your life offering esteem support point out the strengths you overlook when you feel down or unable to complete the treatment. This type of support inspires confidence in yourself due to the amount of confidence your support system offers you. Esteem social support also leads to your believing that you can accomplish anything ones you put your mind to it.

Emotional support: This is the type of support that comprises of physical comfort like constant pats on the back, hugs, empathizing, or simply listening. Emotional support helps you receive big hugs, listening ears, and advice from friends, family, and people who understand what you are going through. You can also receive emotional support from a group of people undergoing the same treatment or people who have succeeded in curing binge eating disorder or emotional eating. Listening to advice from people who have been through the same experiences as yourself, makes it easy for you to continue with the treatment despite the odds.

Tangible support: Tangible support involves taking on certain responsibilities for somebody else to help them deal with problems they are experiencing. In other words, tangible support is simply taking an active role in assisting someone deal with the challenges they are dealing with when undergoing treatment. For instance, your family can help you prep your meals to avoid eating unhealthy foods that can result in a relapse.

Informational support: Informational support is simply offering advice, gathering information, and sharing the results based on what an individual requires. This type of support is essential as it helps you learn what to do every step of the way. For individuals recovering from an eating disorder, your informational support should always be your doctor or therapist.

Remember; always be honest with your support network, as this will help make your journey easy and more achievable.

6. Manage your triggers

When trying to cure an eating disorder it is important to set yourself up for an accomplishment by ensuring you do not expose yourself to unhealthy foods that can cause you to relapse. The first step in accomplishing this is by knowing your triggers. Identifying your triggers is a necessary requirement for individuals undergoing treatment for eating disorders. How do you identify your triggers?

- Start by examining your eating habits. When examining your eating habits ensure that you identify the feelings that cause you to eat even when you are not hungry. Once you recognize those feelings, it is important to try to identify the emotion you are trying to create or avoid with food.

- Take a paper and a piece of paper and record each of the emotions you are trying to create or avoid. Documenting each of these emotions makes it easy to identify when your turn to food to create an emotion or avoid it.

• Next, try to recall what happened the last time you experienced a binging episode or tried to eat your emotions. Recalling the emotions you experienced enables you to learn what causes you to turn to comfort. It also helps you identify when you are most vulnerable to relapses.

• In that piece of paper, create two columns. The first column is an emotions column while the second one is a response column. In the first column, try to identify the emotions that cause a trigger reaction to food. On the second column, try to write down the responses you have to the emotions you experience. For instance, perhaps you got angry and your immediate response to this emotion was eating a large bag of chips. Whatever your response was, ensure that you note it down.

• If you have responses that are repetitive, then now you know what triggers you to binge eat or eat your emotions.

How do you manage your triggers?

As I mentioned earlier, recognizing your triggers is the first step of managing your triggers. Identifying your triggers helps you learn various ways to help you cope with them rather than turn to food for solace. You can do this by incorporating activities you enjoy doing or talking to a therapist to deal with the various issues.

- Accept your feeling even the negative ones. This will help you feel more and learn how to deal with these emotions.

- Keeping a food journal is also another way that can help you manage your triggers. A food diary will help you keep track of what you eat when you eat, the amount of food you consume, and why you eat. This will enable you to separate your emotional hunger from your physical hunger and recognize when your unhealthy eating habits are starting up again.

- Try to practice mindful eating. This is possible by eating with no distractions, as this will help you appreciate the food, its taste, and smell. You should also take smaller bites and eat slowly as this will help you feel fuller.

• Make sure you re-organize your environment to keep you from overeating, like meal planning, having healthy snacks to avoid eating unhealthy snacks, and portion control.

• Listening to your body can also help you develop awareness of your satiety and hunger cues.

• Try to incorporate exercise as part of your daily routine. Exercise will help keep you distracted from the negative emotions. It will also help boost your confidence.

• Also, ensure that your diets are well balanced, as this will help reduce your cravings and rebalance your body's functionality.

• Ensure that you keep unhealthy foods out of your fridge and pantry. This will keep you from a relapse.

7. Seek professional help

I understand how scary it is to realize that you no longer have control over your eating habits despite following the treatment to the letter. However, it is essential to remember that the help you require to get back on the right path is just an email or phone call away. Seeking professional help is important as it helps you deal with the relapse. It also increases your likelihood of recovering from an eating disorder. There is a variety of help available for you from professionals. They are always available to help you recover as well as get back up from a relapse.

How to recognize when you require professional help

Relapse includes mental and behavior changes, which cause one to revert back to unhealthy eating habits. It can also include thoughts that focus too much on your weight, diet or counting calories. This can cause you to excessively worry about the loss of self-control. It is important to understand that there is a high likelihood for people who have struggled with eating disorders for a long time to have numerous relapses.

Another aspect to consider when it comes eating disorder relapses is that your relapse rate will vary depending on the treatment you receive, your age, your interpersonal interactions, and your eating disorder habits. Relapsing does not mean that you have failed in binge eating or emotional eating recovery. It is simply a step that helps you learn how to cope with the numerous challenges you face on the road to recovery. Always remember, that you get through a relapse. Seeking professional enables you to acquire the help you so badly need.

What type of treatment do you require?

The one question people ask quite a lot is what type of professional help should I look for. Should I go to a therapist? Or should visit my doctor? The answers to these questions depend on the nature of your relapses. For instance, if you relapsed due to the amount of pressure you have from friends, family and your environment, then it would be wise to visit a therapist to help you deal with these issues.

If your relapse was due to a lack of specific food in your meal, then talking to your doctor is the best approach to take. Your doctor will help you come up with an inclusive meal plan. This makes it possible to avoid unhealthy foods and manage your cravings.

8. Strive for consistency and not perfection

When recovering from an eating disorder it is essential to realize that, it will take months for you to stop emotional eating or binge eating habits. Your recovery will require work and effort. Changing your eating behaviors is not going to happen overnight but with consistency, it becomes easier to practice. Hence, striving for consistency and not perfection helps in ensuring you do not relapse. People who strive for perfection try to ensure they do not slip-up along the way and this increases room for failure. While people who strive for consistency, understand that there will be slip-ups along the way, but they do not allow their failures to define their recovery. Here are a few tips to help you remain consistent.

Start slowly and gradually progress: A majority of people make the mistake of beginning their recovery process with a high intensity and this may make it impossible for them to keep up after some time. Changing your diet and unhealthy eating habits within a single day or one week is something impossible to do. Therefore, it is essential for you to start by changing one aspect at a time and then gradually increasing the changes.

Accountability: It is quite easy to relapse back to your previous unhealthy eating habits when you have no one to hold you accountable. You may end up eating that bar of chocolate simply because no one will reprimand you for making that choice. However, feeding your cravings when trying to recover from binge eating disorder will cause a derail in your treatment. Having an accountability partner will help you stick to your treatment and nutrition plan and work hard to recover from binge eating disorder or emotional eating.

Do not depend on motivation: Motivation is important but it is short lived especially when undergoing months of treatment for an eating disorder. After weeks of being motivated to stick to your treatment, you may start feeling demotivated and this can cause you to relapse. Therefore, to prevent a relapse from happening, make healthy eating habits a constant practice. The more you stick to your treatment and nutrition plan, the easier it becomes to do it even without motivation.

Develop small habits: Developing habits that seem insignificant when treating an eating disorder is an essential part of being consistent with your treatment.

Some of these small habits include drinking eight glasses of water on a daily basis, avoiding junk food, and exercising for 30 minutes daily among others. Developing these habits is difficult at first but it ends up becoming easier with regular practice.

Set and achieve short-term goals: Recovering from an eating disorder often takes months to accomplish. Therefore, setting short-term goals that will help make your recovery process makes it easy for you to accomplish each goal without having to worry about the long-term goals. You can also set-up a reward system that allows you to reward yourself once you achieve a certain short-term goal.

Relapses are part of your treatment journey do not give up even when you experience a slip-up. You have what it takes to stick to your recovery process. With the above tips, you can achieve the success you want and prevent relapses from occurring.

Conclusion

You do not need this book to tell you that binge eating is having a severely negative effect on your life. This book is here to help you cope with the effects of binging and to help you begin healing from the damage it has caused. Life does not have to be this hard; it does not have to be so difficult just to get through the day. The good news is that you can heal; just reading this book goes to show that you are capable and willing to start on your road to recovery. So no matter what happens, whatever doubts may cross your mind or how many times you may relapse, you can keep going and you will recover. There is a healthy life awaiting you that you deserve. Now you just have to begin walking towards it.